CONTENTS

ENVIRONMENTAL HEALTH CRITERIA FOR DICHLORVOS

WHO TASK GROUP ON DICHLORVOS

Members

Dr L. Albert, Environmental Pollution Programme, National Institute of Biological Resource Research, Veracruz, Mexico

Dr E. Budd, Office of Pesticide Programs, US Environmental Protection Agency, Washington DC, USA

Mr T.P. Bwititi, Ministry of Health, Causeway, Harare, Zimbabwe

Dr S. Deema, Ministry of Agriculture and Cooperatives, Bangkok, Thailand

Dr I. Desi, Department of Hygiene and Epidemiology, Szeged University Medical School, Szeged, Hungary

Dr A.K.H. El Sebae, Pesticides Division, Faculty of Agriculture, Alexandria University, Alexandria, Egypt

Dr R. Goulding, Keats House, Guy's Hospital, London, United Kingdom (*Chairman*)

Dr J. Jeyaratnam, National University of Singapore, Department of Social Medicine and Public Health, Faculty of Medicine, National University Hospital, Singapore (*Vice-Chairman*)

Dr Y. Osman, Occupational Health Department, Ministry of Health, Khartoum, Sudan

Dr A. Takanaka, Division of Pharmacology, National Institute of Hygienic Sciences, Tokyo, Japan

Observers

Dr N. Punja, European Chemical Industry, Ecology and Toxicology Centre (ECETOC), Brussels, Belgium

Ms J. Shaw, International Group of National Associations of Manufacturers of Agrochemical Products (GIFAP), Brussels, Belgium

Secretariat

Dr M. Gilbert, International Register of Potentially Toxic Chemicals, United Nations Environment Programme, Geneva, Switzerland

Dr K.W. Jager, International Programme on Chemical Safety, World Health Organization, Geneva, Switzerland (*Secretary*)

Dr T. Ng, Office of Occupational Health, World Health Organization, Geneva, Switzerland

Dr G. Quélennec, Pesticides Development and Safe Use Unit, World Health Organization, Geneva, Switzerland

Dr R.C. Tincknell, Beaconsfield, Buckinghamshire, United Kingdom (*Temporary Adviser*)

Dr G.J. Van Esch, Bilthoven, Netherlands (*Temporary Adviser) (Co-Rapporteur*)

Dr E.A.H. Van Heemstra-Lequin, Laren, Netherlands (*Temporary Adviser) (Co-Rapporteur*)

NOTE TO READERS OF THE CRITERIA DOCUMENTS

Every effort has been made to present information in the criteria documents as accurately as possible without unduly delaying their publication. In the interest of all users of the environmental health criteria documents, readers are kindly requested to communicate any errors that may have occurred to the Manager of the International Programme on Chemical Safety, World Health Organization, Geneva, Switzerland, in order that they may be included in corrigenda, which will appear in subsequent volumes.

* * *

A detailed data profile and a legal file can be obtained from the International Register of Potentially Toxic Chemicals, Palais des Nations, 1211 Geneva 10, Switzerland (Telephone no. 988400 - 985850).

ENVIRONMENTAL HEALTH CRITERIA FOR DICHLORVOS

A WHO Task Group on Environmental Health Criteria for Dichlorvos met in Geneva from 1 to 5 December 1986. Dr M. Mercier, Manager, IPCS, opened the meeting and welcomed the participants on behalf of the heads of the three IPCS co-sponsoring organizations (UNEP/ILO/WHO). The Group reviewed and revised the draft criteria document and made an evaluation of the risks for human health and the environment from exposure to dichlorvos.

The drafts of the document were prepared by DR E.A.H. VAN HEEMSTRA-LEQUIN and DR G.J. VAN ESCH of the Netherlands.

Draft summaries of Japanese studies on dichlorvos were prepared and finalized by DR M. ETO (Kyushu University), and DR J. MIYAMOTO and DR M. MATSUO (Sumitomo Chemical Co., Ltd), with the assistance of the staff of the NATIONAL INSTITUTE OF HYGIENIC SCIENCES, Tokyo, Japan and DR I. YAMAMOTO (Tokyo University of Agriculture).

The proprietary data mentioned in the document were made available to the Central Unit of the IPCS by Temana International Ltd, Richmond, United Kingdom for evaluation by the Task Group.

The efforts of all who helped in the preparation and finalization of the document are gratefully acknowledged.

* * *

The proprietary information contained in this document cannot replace documentation for registration purposes, because the latter has to be closely linked to the source, the manufacturing route, and the purity/impurities of the substance to be registered. The data should be used in accordance with paragraphs 82-84 and recommendation paragraph 90 of the 2nd FAO Government Consultation (FAO, 1982).

* * *

Partial financial support for the publication of this criteria document was kindly provided by the United States Department of Health and Human Services, through a contract from the National Institute of Environmental Health Sciences, Research Triangle Park, North Carolina, USA - a WHO Collaborating Centre for Environmental Health Effects. The United Kingdom Department of Health and Social Security generously supported the cost of printing.

1. SUMMARY AND RECOMMENDATIONS

1.1 General

Dichlorvos, an organophosphate, is a direct-acting cholinesterase (ChE)[a] inhibitor. Since 1961, it has been commercially manufactured and used throughout the world as a contact and stomach insecticide. It is used to protect stored products and crops (mainly in greenhouses), and to control internal and external parasites in livestock (granules of impregnated resin) and insects in houses, buildings, aircraft, and outdoor areas (as aerosols, liquid sprays, or impregnated cellulosic, ceramic, or resin strips). The present worldwide production of dichlorvos is about 4 million kg per year.

The purity of the technical grade product is at least 97%, and the type of impurities depends on the manufacturing process. In the presence of moisture, dichlorvos breaks down to form acidic products that are eventually mineralized. Technical dichlorvos may be stabilized, which improves the storage stability, but it is not normally necessary to stabilize high purity products. In the past, 2 - 4% epichlorohydrin has been used for this purpose. Dichlorvos is soluble in water and miscible with most organic solvents and aerosol propellants. The vapour pressure of dichlorvos is relatively high (1.6 Pa at 20 °C).

Methods for sampling and analysing dichlorvos in food, feed, and the environment and for determining the inhibition of ChE activity in blood, red blood cells, plasma, and brain are described.

1.2 Environmental Transport, Distribution, and Transformation

Dichlorvos is not directly applied to soil, but is added to water to control invertebrate fish parasites encountered during intensive fish farming. It breaks down rapidly in humid air, water, and soil, both by abiotic and biotic processes, whereas on wooden surfaces it may persist for a longer time (39% remaining after 33 days). It degrades mainly to dichloro-ethanol, dichloroacetaldehyde (DCA), dichloroacetic acid, dimethylphosphate, dimethylphosphoric acid, and other water-soluble compounds, which are eventually mineralized.

Dichlorvos is rapidly lost from leaf surfaces by volatilization and hydrolysis.

Accidental spillage of dichlorvos may have acute hazardous effects on man and the environment. However, long-term effects are unlikely, in view of the volatility and instability in humid environments. Bioaccumulation or biomagnification do not occur.

---

[a] Cholinesterase is the enzyme which breaks down acetylcholine (ACh), the transmitter at cholinergic nerve synapses.

1.3 Environmental Levels and Human Exposure

The indoor air dichlorvos concentrations resulting from household and public health use depend on the method of application, temperature, and humidity. For example, one impregnated resin strip per 30 m^3 results in concentrations of the order of 0.1 - 0.3 mg/m^3 the first week (the latter only in special circumstances), subsequently decreasing to 0.02 mg/m^3 or less over the next few weeks.

Dichlorvos residues in food commodities are generally low and are readily destroyed during processing. The metabolite DCA may also be present in detectable amounts. Total-diet studies in the United Kingdom and the USA have confirmed that no, or very little, dichlorvos is found in prepared meals.

Exposure of the general population via food and drinking-water as a result of agricultural or post-harvest use of dichlorvos is negligible. However, household and public health use do give rise to exposure, principally through inhalation and dermal absorption.

Similar routes of exposure occur in professional pest control with dichlorvos. In warehouses, mushroom houses, and greenhouses, the concentrations of dichlorvos in the air are in general below 1 mg/m^3 when the recommended application rates are used, but in certain circumstances they may rise considerably above this level.

1.4 Kinetics and Metabolism

Dichlorvos is readily absorbed via all routes of exposure. After oral administration, it is metabolized in the liver before it reaches the systemic circulation.

One hour after the oral administration of ^{32}P-dichlorvos, maximum concentrations of radioactivity are found in the kidneys, liver, stomach, and intestines. In bone, the increase is slower, due to inorganic phosphate entering the phosphate pool of the organism.

Pigs administered a single oral dose of ^{14}C-labelled dichlorvos as a slow-release polyvinyl chloride (PVC) formulation, showed radioactivity in all tissues, the highest level being in the liver after 2 days, and the lowest being in the brain. Pregnant sows were fed vinyl-1-^{14}C-dichlorvos or ^{36}Cl-dichlorvos in PVC pellets at 4 mg dichlorvos/kg body weight per day during the last third of the gestation period. Although the tissues of the sows and piglets contained ^{14}C or ^{36}Cl ranging from 0.3 to 18 mg/kg tissue, no radioactivity was associated with dichlorvos or its primary metabolites.

Up to 70% of the dichlorvos inhaled by pigs is taken up into the body. When rats and mice inhaled dichlorvos (90 mg/m^3 for 4 h), none or very little (up to 0.2 mg/kg) was found in blood, liver, testes, lung, or brain. The highest concentrations (up to 2.4 mg/kg tissue) were found in kidneys and adipose tissue. Dichlorvos rapidly disappeared from the kidneys with a half-life of approximately 14 min.

Dichlorvos is metabolized mainly in the liver via 2 enzymatic pathways: one, producing desmethyldichlorvos, is glutathione dependent, while the other, resulting in dimethyl-phosphate and DCA, is glutathione independent. The metabolism of dichlorvos in various species, including man, is rapid and uses similar pathways. Differences between species relate to the rate of metabolism rather than to a difference of metabolites.

The major route of metabolism of the vinyl portion of dichlorvos leads to (a) dichloroethanol glucuronide and (b) hippuric acid, urea, carbon dioxide, and other endogenous chemicals, such as glycine and serine, which give rise to high levels of radioactivity in the tissues. No evidence of the accumulation of dichlorvos or potentially toxic metabolites has been found.

The major route for the elimination of the phosphorus-containing moiety is via the urine, with expired air being a less important route. However, the vinyl moiety is mainly eliminated in the expired air, and less so in the urine. In cows, elimination is roughly equally distributed between urine and faeces.

1.5 Effects on Organisms in the Environment

The effect of dichlorvos on microorganisms is variable and species dependent. Certain microorganisms have the ability to metabolize dichlorvos but the pesticide may interfere with the endogenous oxidative metabolism of the organism. In certain organisms it causes growth inhibition, while in others it has no influence or may even stimulate growth. Dichlorvos has little or no toxic effect on microorganisms degrading organic matter in sewage. The above effects have been seen over the wide dose range of 0.1 - 100 mg/litre.

The acute toxicity of dichlorvos for both freshwater and estuarine species of fish is moderate to high (96-h LC_{50} values range from 0.2 to approximately 10 mg/litre). Brain and liver ChE inhibition in certain fish was found at dose levels of 0.25 - 1.25 mg/litre, but recovery of ChE activity took place when they were returned to clean water.

Invertebrates are more sensitive to dichlorvos. Levels above 0.05 μg/litre may have deleterious effects. Dichlorvos also has a high oral toxicity for birds. The LD_{50} values are in the range of 5 - 40 mg/kg body weight. In short-term dietary studies, the compound was slightly to moderately toxic for birds. Brain ChE inhibition was seen at 50 mg/kg diet or more and at 500 mg/kg diet, half of the birds died. There have been instances when chickens and ducks have died after accidental access to dichlorvos-contaminated feed and drinking-water.

Dichlorvos is highly toxic for honey bees. The LD_{50} by oral administration is 0.29 μg/g bee, and after topical application is 0.65 μg/g bee.

1.6 Effects on Experimental Animals and *In Vitro* Test Systems

Dichlorvos is moderately to highly toxic when administered in single doses to a variety of animal species by several routes. It directly inhibits acetylcholinesterase (AChE) activity in the nervous system and in other tissues. Maximum inhibition generally occurs within 1 h, and is followed by rapid recovery. The oral LD_{50} for the rat is 30 - 110 mg/kg body weight, depending on the solvent used. The hazard classification of dichlorvos by WHO (1986a) is based on an oral LD_{50} for the rat of 56 mg/kg body weight. The signs of intoxication are typical of organophosphorus poisoning, i.e., salivation, lachrymation, diarrhoea, tremors, and terminal convulsions, with death occurring from respiratory failure. The signs of intoxication are usually apparent shortly after dosing, and, at lethal doses, death occurs within 1 h. Survivors recover completely within 24 h.

Potentiation is slight when dichlorvos is given orally in combination with other organophosphates, but in combination with malathion it is marked.

In short-term toxicity studies on the mouse, rat, dog, pig, and monkey, inhibition of plasma, red blood cell, and brain ChE are the most important signs of toxicity. After oral administration, approximately 0.5 mg/kg body weight (range, 0.3 - 0.7 mg/kg) did not produce ChE inhibition. In a 2-year study on dogs, ChE inhibition was noted at 3.2 mg/kg body weight or more.

Flea collar dermatitis has been described in dogs and cats wearing dichlorvos-impregnated PVC flea collars. This was a primary irritant contact dermatitis which may have been caused by dichlorvos.

Many short-term inhalation studies on different animal species have been carried out. Air concentrations in the range of 0.2 - 1 mg/m^3 do not affect ChE activity significantly. Other effects, such as growth inhibition and increase in liver weight have been reported at dose levels at least 10 - 20 times higher.

It is possible to produce clinical neuropathy in hens, but the doses of dichlorvos required are far in excess of the LD_{50}. The effects are associated with high inhibition of neurotoxic esterase (NTE) in the brain and spinal cord. In the rat, however, neuropathic changes in the white matter of the brain have been reported following repeated daily oral application of an LD_{50} dose.

Immune suppression has been reported in rabbits. At present, no evaluation as to the relevance for human beings can be given; more attention to this aspect is needed.

In a long-term study, rats fed dichlorvos in the diet for 2 years showed no signs of intoxication. Hepatocellular fatty vacuolization of the liver and ChE inhibition were significant at the two highest dose levels (2.5 and 12.5 mg/kg body weight).

In a carefully conducted long-term inhalation study on rats with whole body exposure (23 h/day, for 2 years), results were comparable with those seen in the oral study. No effects were seen at 0.05 mg/m^3; inhibition of ChE activity took place at 0.48 mg/m^3 or more.

In several reproduction studies on rats and domestic animals, no effects were seen on reproduction, and there was no embryotoxicity at dose levels that did not cause maternal toxicity. At toxic doses, dichlorvos may cause reversible disturbances of spermatogenesis in mice and rats. It was not teratogenic in several studies carried out on rats and rabbits.

Dichlorvos is an alkylating agent and binds *in vitro* to bacterial and mammalian nucleic acids. It is mutagenic in a number of microbial systems, but there is no evidence of mutagenicity in intact mammals, where it is rapidly degraded by esterases in blood and other tissues.

Dichlorvos carcinogenicity has been investigated in mice (oral studies) and rats (oral and inhalation studies). The dose levels used in 2-year oral studies were up to 800 mg/litre drinking-water or 600 mg/kg diet for mice, and up to 280 mg/litre drinking-water or 234 mg/kg diet for rats. In a rat inhalation study, dichlorvos concentrations in air of up to 4.7 mg/m^3 were tested for 2 years. No statistically significant increase in tumour incidence was found. In two recent carcinogenicity studies on mice and rats, dichlorvos was administered by intubation at dose levels between 10 and 40 mg/kg body weight (mice) and 4 and 8 mg/kg body weight (rat) for up to 2 years. Only preliminary information has been provided. The evidence for carcinogenicity in these new studies is difficult to interpret at this time. Only when complete and final reports become available will it be possible to draw more definitive conclusions (in this context, see footnote p. 95, section 8.7.3).

From acute and short-term studies, it is clear that the metabolites of dichlorvos are all less toxic than the parent compound. Only DCA was positive in a few mutagenicity tests.

1.7 Effects on Man

A fatal case of dichlorvos poisoning has been described in the general population: despite correct treatment, a suicide succeeded with approximately 400 mg dichlorvos/kg body weight. In another poisoning case, a woman ingested about 100 mg dichlorvos/kg and survived, following intensive care for 14 days. Two workers who had skin exposure to a concentrated dichlorvos formulation, and failed to wash it off, died of poisoning.

There have been two clinical reports describing four patients suffering from severe poisoning from dichlorvos, taken orally, who survived after treatment and who showed delayed neurotoxic effects. Thus although the possibility of neuropathy in man cannot be excluded, it is likely to occur only after almost lethal oral doses.

Since the 1960s, field studies in malaria control have been carried out and the interiors of aircraft have been sprayed with dichlorvos. Exposure to concentrations in the air of up to 0.5 mg/m^3 were without clinical effects, and no, or only insignificant, inhibition of blood ChE activity was noted.

When dichlorvos was administered orally to human volunteers (single or repeated doses of a slow-release PVC formulation), significant inhibition of red blood cell ChE activity was found at 4 mg/kg body weight or more. At 1 mg/kg body weight or more, plasma ChE activity was significantly inhibited. Daily oral doses of 2 mg dichlorvos/person for 28 days reduced plasma ChE activity by 30%, but red cell ChE activity was unaffected.

Human volunteers who were exposed to dichlorvos by inhalation for a certain period per day for a number of consecutive days or weeks showed ChE inhibition at a concentration of 1 mg/m^3 or more, but not at 0.5 mg/m^3. These results were confirmed in studies with pesticide operators who came into contact with dichlorvos.

Hospitalized patients showed similar results after oral administration or exposure by inhalation. Sick adults and children and healthy pregnant women and babies in hospital wards treated with dichlorvos strips (1 strip/30 or 40 m^3) displayed normal ChE activity. Only subjects exposed 24 h/day to concentrations above 0.1 mg/m^3 or patients with liver insufficiency showed a moderate decrease in plasma ChE activity.

No significant effects on plasma or red blood cell ChE activity were observed in people exposed to the recommended rate of one dichlorvos strip per 30 m^3 in their homes over a period of 6 months, even when the strips were replaced at shorter intervals than that normally recommended. The maximum average concentration in the air was approximately 0.1 mg/m^3.

In factory workers exposed to an average of 0.7 mg/m^3 for 8 months, significant inhibition of plasma and red blood cell ChE activity was found.

Cases of dermatitis and skin sensitization due to dichlorvos have been described in workers handling and spraying different types of pesticides. In addition cross-sensitization with certain pesticides has been seen.

2. IDENTITY, PHYSICAL AND CHEMICAL PROPERTIES, ANALYTICAL METHODS

2.1 Identity

Primary constituent

Chemical structure:	$Cl_2C{=}CHO\overset{O}{\overset{\|}{P}}(OCH_3)_2$
Chemical formula:	$C_4H_7Cl_2O_4P$
Chemical names:	2,2-dichloroethenyl dimethylphosphate (CAS); 2,2-dichlorovinyl dimethylphosphate (IUPAC)
Common synonyms:	Bayer-19149, DDVF, DDVP, ENT-20738, OMS-14, SD 1750, C-177
CAS registry number:	62-73-7

Technical product

Common trade names:	Dedevap, Nogos, Nuvan, Phosvit, Vapona[a]
Purity:	should not be less than 97% (WHO, 1985)
Impurities:	depend on the manufacturing process (section 3.2.1.2)
Additives:	In the presence of traces of moisture, dichlorvos slowly breaks down to form acidic products that catalyse further decomposition of the compound. In the past, 2 - 4% epichlorohydrin was added to stabilize the technical grade product (Melnikov, 1971). Other stabilizers may now be used in some products, but improved technology and purity has largely eliminated the need for stabilizers.

---

a The Shell trademark Vapona was formerly used exclusively for dichlorvos and dichlorvos-containing formulations. More recently, this trademark has been used more widely to include formulations containing other active ingredients.

2.2 Physical and Chemical Properties

Dichlorvos is a colourless to amber liquid with an aromatic odour.

Some physical and chemical properties of dichlorvos are given in Table 1.

Table 1. Some physical and chemical properties of dichlorvos[a]

Relative molecular mass	221
Boiling point	35 °C at 6.7 Pa (0.05 mmHg); 74 °C at 133 Pa (1 mmHg)[b]
Vapour pressure (20 °C)	1.6 Pa ($1.2 \cdot 10^{-2}$ mmHg)
Density (25 °C)	1.415
Refractive index	$N_D^{25} = 1.4523$
Solubility	about 10 g/litre water at 20 °C; 2 - 3 g/kg kerosene; miscible with most organic solvents and aerosol propellants
Stability	dichlorvos is stable to heat but is hydrolysed by water; a saturated aqueous solution at room temperature is converted to dimethylphosphate and dichloroacetaldehyde at a rate of about 3% per day, more rapidly in alkali
Corrosivity	corrosive to iron and mild steel
Log *n*-octanol/water partition coefficient	1.47[c]

[a] From: Worthing & Walker (1983).
[b] From: Melnikov (1971).
[c] From: Bowman & Sans (1983).

2.3 Conversion Factors

1 ppm = 10 mg/m^3 at 25 °C and 101 kPa (760 mmHg);

1 mg/m^3 = 0.1 ppm

2.4 Analytical Methods

The various analytical methods are summarized in Tables 2, 3, 4, and 5.

Table 2. Analytical methods for dichlorvos residues in food and biological media recommended by the Codex Working Group on Methods of Analysis

Sample	Extraction	Clean-up	Detection and quantification	Recovery	Limit of detection	Reference
grain	methanol		gas-liquid chromatography with thermionic phosphorus detector or flame photometric phosphorus detector		0.02 mg/kg	Anon. (1973)
cereal products	petroleum ether/ ethyl ether	Florisil column	gas chromatography with flame photometric detector or thermionic ionization detector	70 - 80%	0.0025 mg/kg	Mestres et al. (1979b)
cereals	hexane hexane/acetonitrile benzene	activated charcoal column extraction acetone/hexane	gas chromatography with flame photometric detection	72 - 83%	0.01 ng (sensitivity)	Aoki et al. (1975)
crops	dichloromethane or ethylacetate	steam distillation	gas-liquid chromatography with flame photometric detector, thermionic ionization detector, or electron capture detector	80 - 100%	0.01 mg/kg	Elgar et al. (1970)
	ethylacetate/ dichloromethane	Florisil column	gas chromatography with flame photometric detector	80%	0.002 - 0.05 mg/kg	Mestres et al. (1979a)

Table 2 (contd).

Sample	Extraction	Clean-up	Detection and quantification	Recovery	Limit of detection	Reference
fruit and vegetables	acetonitrile	extraction with chloroform; residue in acetone	gas-liquid chromatography with flame photometric detector or thermionic ionization detector	approximately 90% (at 0.5 mg/kg)		Anon. (1977)
onions	acetonitrile benzene	amberlite XAD-8 column benzene/ dichloromethane	gas chromatography with flame photo metric detection	82%		Iwata et al. (1981)
	chloroform, methanol	HCl and Celite	gas-liquid chromatography with thermionic ionization detector	approximately 90% (at 0.05 - 0.5 mg/kg)	0.01 mg/kg	Krause & Kirchhoff (1970)
	acetone and partition with petroleum ether and dichloromethane	double concentration with petroleum ether	gas-liquid chromatography with flame photometric detector	90% (at 0.1 mg/kg)		Luke et al. (1981)
eggplant fruit	water/methanol ether/petroleum ether		gas chromatography with flame photometric detection	95%	0.004 mg	Nakamura & Shiba (1980)

Table 2 (contd).

plants	methanol	ether/petroleum ether	gas-liquid chromatography with phosphorus detector	95 - 100%	0.1 mg/kg	Dräger (1968)
	acetonitrile or dichloromethane or methanol/chloroform	liquid-liquid partitioning none none	thin-layer chromatography enzymatic assay using: bee head extract pig liver extract beef liver extract		indo-phenyl-acetate / bromo-indoxyl-acetate 5 ng / - 5 ng / 1 ng 5 ng / 0.1 ng	Mendoza & Shields (1971)
	acetone or dichloromethane	column chromatography	thin-layer chromatography enzymatic assay (horse serum)		1 - 2 ng	Ambrus et al. (1981)
		without clean-up	thin-layer chromatography silver nitrate + UV		100 ng	
			gas-liquid chromatography with thermionic ionization detector or electron capture detector	55 - 80%	0.1 - 1 ng 0.01 - 0.05 ng typical limit of detection 0.005 - 0.02 mg/kg	
vegetable and animal food, tobacco	acetone; dichloromethane or acetonitrile; dichloromethane	sweep co-distillation	gas chromatography with thermionic phosphorus detector	75 - 100% (at 0.03 - 0.5 mg/kg)		Eichner (1978)

Table 2 (contd).

Sample	Extraction	Clean-up	Detection and quantification	Recovery	Limit of detection	Reference
whole meal	cereal: methanol; fats: hexane and acetonitrile; others: acetonitrile	depending on type of sample	gas-liquid chromatography with thermionic phosphorus detector, caesium bromide tips			Abbott et al. (1970)
	homogenized sample, ethyl acetate - hexane and HCl	silica gel column; elution with acetone/hexane	gas chromatography with flame photometric detector	97 - 100%	0.005 mg/kg (sensitivity)	Dale et al. (1973)
animal tissues	dichloromethane or ethylacetate	steam distillation	gas-liquid chromatography with flame photometric detector, thermionic ionization detector, or electron capture detector	80 - 100%	0.01 mg/kg	Elgar et al. (1970)
milk	methanol	acetonitrile and ether/petroleum ether	gas chromatography with phosphorus detector	80 - 90% (at 0.01 - 0.1 mg/kg)	0.01 mg/kg	Dräger (1968)
	acetonitrile	dichloromethane; methane; residue dissolved in acetone	gas-liquid chromatography with thermionic phosphorus detector, caesium bromide tips			Abbott et al. (1970)

Table 3. Other analytical methods for dichlorvos residues in food and biological media

Sample	Extraction	Clean-up	Detection and quantification	Recovery	Limit of detection	Reference
agricultural crops, animal tissues, beverages, food	ethyl acetate	none except for oil extracts	gas-liqud chromatography with phosphorus detector		food, crops: 0.02 mg/kg	Anon. (1972)
fruit, vegetables	hexane/acetone	aluminium oxide column	thin-layer chromatography; nitrobenzylpyridine/triaza undecamethylene diamine			Wood & Kanagasabapathy (1983)
organs/ tissues;	ethanol	none	thin-layer chromatography enzymatic assay (beef liver)		0.2 ng	Ackerman et al. (1969)
contents of stomach, intestines; urine	none or chloroform	none				
milk,	dichloromethane	silica gel column, mixed solvents	gas chromatography with flame photometric detector	95%	0.003 mg/kg	Ivey & Claborn (1969)

Table 3 (contd).

Sample	Extraction	Clean-up	Detection and quantification	Recovery	Limit of detection	Reference
fat, chicken, skin,	hexane			80%	0.002 mg/kg	Ivey & Claborn (1969)
muscle, eggs	acetonitrile	silica gel column		80%	0.002 mg/kg	Ivey & Claborn (1969)
animal tissues[a] and fluids	depending on sample	only for fat tissues	gas-liquid chromatography with phosphorus detector		0.05 - 0.1 mg/kg	Schultz et al. (1971)
milk		silica gel column; alkaline hydrolysis and condensation with *o*-phenylenediamine	polarography	85%	0.15 mg/kg	Davidek et al. (1976)

[a] Methods for analysing residues of four metabolites of dichlorvos are also given.

Table 4. Analytical methods for determining the dichlorvos concentration and ChE activity in blood

Sample	Extraction	Clean-up	Detection and quantification	Recovery	Limit of detection	Reference
<u>Dichlorvos concentrations</u>						
blood	acetonitrile hexane		gas chromatography with flame photometric detector	86%		Ivey & Claborn (1969)
blood/serum	chloroform	none	thin-layer chromatography enzymatic assay (beef liver)			Ackerman et al. (1969)
blood[a]	water/ethanol extracted with ethyl acetate	none	gas-liquid chromatography with phosphorus detector			Schultz et al. (1971); Anon. (1972)
<u>ChE activity</u>						
blood (plasma and red cell)			electrometric method for ChE activity, release of acetic acid from ACh; pH change			Michel (1949)
whole blood ChE	ACh-perchlorate and bromothymol blue		tintometric method			Edson (1958)

Table 4 (contd).

Sample	Extraction	Clean-up	Detection and quantification	Recovery	Limit of detection	Reference
ChE activity (contd).						
whole blood and plasma ChE	dithiobis-nitro-benzoic acid (DTNB) + acetylthiocholine (animal blood) or propionyl thiocholine (human blood); eserine salicylate (esterase inhibitor)		colorimetry at 420 nm			Voss & Sachsse (1970)
whole blood and erythrocyte ChE	DTNB + acetylthiocholine iodide		spectrophotometry at 412 nm			Ellman et al. (1961); Anderson et al. (1978)
whole blood and erythrocyte ChE	dithiodipyridine (DTPD) + propionyl thiocholine; esterase inhibitor		spectrophotometry at 324 nm			Augustinsson et al. (1978)

a Methods for analysing concentrations of four metabolites of dichlorvos are also given.

Table 5. Analytical methods for the determination of dichlorvos in air, soil, and water

Sample	Extraction	Clean-up	Detection and quantification	Recovery	Limit of detection	Reference
<u>Air</u>						
glass tubes containing:						
water			electrometric pH method			Elgar & Steer (1972)
ethyl acetate	none		gas-liquid chromatography with phosphorus detector		0.01 mg/m^3	Anon. (1972)
potassium nitrate	elution with hexane		gas chromatography with flame photometric detector	80%		Bryant & Minett (1978)
XAD-2 (personal sampling)	desorption with toluene		gas chromatography with flame photometric phosphorus detector		0.2 µg	NIOSH (1979); Gunderson (1981)
<u>Soil</u>						
soil	acetone	column chromatography	thin-layer chromatography enzymatic assay (horse serum)		1 - 2 ng	Ambrus et al. (1981)

Table 5 (contd).

Sample	Extraction	Clean-up	Detection and quantification	Recovery	Limit of detection	Reference
soil		without clean-up	thin-layer chromatography; silver nitrate + UV		100 ng	Ambrus et al. (1981)
soil	ether/acetone (7:3) petroleum ether		flame photometric detector-gas chromatography	91%	5 μg	Goto (1977)
Water						
water	dichloromethane	column chromatography	thin-layer chromatography enzymatic assay (horse serum)		1 - 2 ng	Ambrus et al. (1981)
		without clean-up	thin-layer chromatography; silver nitrate + UV		100 ng	
			gas-liquid chromatography with electron capture detector or thermionic ionization detector	55 - 70%	0.01 - 0.05 ng; 0.1 - 1 ng typical limit of detection 0.0001 mg/kg	

2.4.1 Sampling methods

2.4.1.1 Food and feed

The "Codex Recommended Method of Sampling for the Determination of Pesticide Residues" (Codex Alimentarius Commission, 1979; GIFAP, 1982) describes sampling rates and acceptance criteria in relation to the analytical sample and the Codex maximum residue limits (Codex Alimentarius Commission, 1983).

2.4.1.2 Blood

Where samples cannot be determined immediately, e.g., samples taken in the field, they must be frozen in order to prevent the reactivation of inhibited plasma ChE or erythrocyte AChE. When freezing facilities are limited, or where samples must be transported and/or stored for several days, samples of whole blood are applied to filter paper. These samples can be stored at room temperature for at least 2 weeks and in a refrigerator for more than 6 weeks without reducing the efficiency of elution from the filter paper (Eriksson & Fayersson, 1980).

2.4.1.3 Air

Methods of sampling air for pesticides have been reviewed by Miles et al. (1970), Van Dijk & Visweswariah (1975), Lewis (1976), and Thomas & Nishioka (1985).

Miles et al. (1970) compared the widely-used techniques and came to the conclusion that, although each method has certain advantages, none are ideal. Packed adsorption columns are very efficient for trapping vapours, but recovery of the sample is frequently difficult. Glass fibre filters or cellulose filter pads permit the collection of large volumes of air in short periods of time, but their efficiency for vapours is low, and unknown losses of aerosol samples occur. Membrane filters are good for liquid aerosols and vapours, but the sampling rate is slow. However, Tessari & Spencer (1971) considered collection on a moist nylon net to be the best sampling method for aerosol and vapour-phase pesticides. Freeze-out traps are of limited value in field work. Impingers seem to offer a compromise; they can be operated at quite a fast flow rate, they are efficient for collection of aerosols, and, with correct solvent selection, they collect vapours efficiently.

Heuser & Scudamore (1966) used dry potassium nitrate in an adsorption tube and were able to measure less than 1 $\mu g/m^3$ of dichlorvos in air.

When Miles et al. (1970) used two Greenburg-Smith-type impingers containing water, they trapped up to 97% of dichlorvos. However, when ethylacetate was used instead of water, more than 95% of the available dichlorvos was collected in the first impinger (Anon., 1972).

For personal sampling of dichlorvos in the work environment, Gunderson (1981) collected air samples from the worker's breathing zone in glass tubes packed with XAD-2 (a styrene-divinyl benzene cross-linked porous polymer) as sorbent. A calibrated personal sampling pump drew air through the filter.

2.4.2 Analytical methods

2.4.2.1 Analysis of technical and formulated dichlorvos products

Dichlorvos products can be analysed by gas-liquid chromatography, infrared spectrometry (Oba & Kawabata, 1962), or by reaction with an excess of iodine which is estimated by titration (CIPAC Handbook, 1980). A colorimetric method to estimate dichlorvos in formulations was described by Mitsui et al. (1963) and improved by Ogata et al. (1975). Formulated dichlorvos can be analysed by gas-liquid chromatography after extraction or dilution with chloroform, or after partitioning of the dichlorvos into acetonitrile (Anon., 1972). Heuser & Scudamore (1975) described a method to assess the output of dichlorvos slow-release strips for insect control. A method for the analysis of dichlorvos in technical and formulated products was reported in WHO (1985).

Qualitative methods to identify dichlorvos or to separate and estimate it in the presence of other organophosphorus compounds were described by Sera et al. (1959) and Yamashita (1961).

2.4.2.2 Determination of dichlorvos residues

The main methods for determining dichlorvos are:

(a) thin-layer chromatography (TLC);

(b) enzyme-inhibition detection, coupled with TLC;

(c) gas chromatography (GC) with electron capture detector (ECD) (specificity is poor);

(d) GC with flame photometric detector (FPD) (the most widely-used method for the determination of organophosphorus compounds);

(e) GC with thermionic alkaline flame ionization detector (TID), which is more sensitive to phosphorous-containing compounds than the FPD, but is less stable (Lewis, 1976).

Mendoza (1974) reviewed the applications of the TLC-enzyme-inhibition technique for pesticide residues and metabolite analyses involving determination and confirmation of pesticides.

IUPAC's Commission on Pesticide Chemistry examined simplified analytical methods for screening pesticide residues and their metabolites in food and environmental samples (Batora et al., 1981).

The Codex Committee on Pesticide Residues lists recommended methods for the analysis of dichlorvos (FAO/WHO, 1986).

2.4.2.3 Confirmatory tests

Confirmation of the identity of the residue by an independent test is an essential part of good laboratory practice. The ultimate choice of a confirmatory test depends on the technique used in the initial determination and on the available instrumentation and necessary expertise. Details of various confirmatory tests have been published (Mendoza & Shields, 1971; Shalik et al., 1971; Mestres et al., 1977; Cochrane, 1979).

2.4.2.4 Food

The Working Group on Methods of Analysis of the Codex Committee on Pesticide Residues has produced guidelines on good analytical practice in residue analysis and Recommendations of Methods of Analysis for Pesticide Residues (Codex Alimentarius Commission, 1983). The recommended methods are mostly multiresidue ones and are suitable for analysing as many pesticide product combinations as possible up to the Codex maximum residue limits. The methods are summarized in Table 2. Other methods for residue analysis are given in Table 3.

2.4.2.5 Blood

Methods for analysing dichlorvos concentrations in blood are given in Table 4. The determination of the four metabolites of dichlorvos was described by Schultz et al. (1971).

The most frequently used method for determining ChE activity in blood is that of Ellman et al. (1961), subsequently modified by Voss & Sachsse (1970) and Augustinsson et al. (1978). An improvement of this spectrophotometric method for determining ChE activity in erythrocytes and tissue homogenates was described by Anderson et al. (1978). The method of Ellman et al. (1961) has been developed by WHO (1970) into a field kit for the determination of blood ChE activity.

2.4.2.6 Air

A review of the analysis of airborne pesticides has been published by Lewis (1976). Methods for determining dichlorvos concentrations in air are given in Table 5.

2.4.2.7 Soil and water

Methods are summarized in Table 5.

3. SOURCES OF HUMAN AND ENVIRONMENTAL EXPOSURE

3.1 Natural Occurrence

Dichlorvos does not occur as a natural product.

3.2 Man-Made Sources

3.2.1 Production levels and processes

3.2.1.1 Worldwide production figures

Dichlorvos has been manufactured commercially since 1961 in many countries. Worldwide production figures for 1984 are given in Table 6.

Table 6. The worldwide production of dichlorvos in 1984

Country	Production in tonnes
Eastern Europe	220
Japan	1100
Latin America	400
Middle East (including India and Pakistan)	1200
South-East Asia	500
USA	500
Western Europe	300
Total	4220

Of this total production, 60% is used in plant protection, 30% for public hygiene and vector control, and 10% to protect stored products (GIFAP, personal communication, 1986).

3.2.1.2 Manufacturing processes

Dichlorvos can be manufactured by the dehydrochlorination of trichlorphon (chlorophos) through the action of caustic alkalis in aqueous solution at 40 - 50 °C.

$$(CH_3O)_2\overset{\overset{O}{\|}}{P}CH(OH)CCl_3 + KOH \rightarrow (CH_3O)_2\overset{\overset{O}{\|}}{P}OCH{=}CCl_2 + KCl + H_2O$$

The yield of dichlorvos in this process does not exceed 60%.

Another process is the reaction of chloral with trimethylphosphite:

$$(CH_3O)_3P + CCl_3CHO \rightarrow (CH_3O)_2\overset{O}{\overset{\|}{P}}OCH{=}CCl_2 + CH_3Cl$$

Using this method, dichlorvos of 92 - 93% purity can be produced by either a batch or a continuous process (Melnikov, 1971).

3.2.2 Uses

Dichlorvos is a contact and stomach insecticide with fumigant and penetrant action. It is used for the protection of stored products and crops (mainly greenhouse crops), and for the control of internal and external parasites in livestock and insects in buildings, aircraft, and outdoor areas.

As a household and public health insecticide with fumigant action, dichlorvos has widespread use in the form of aerosol or liquid sprays, or as impregnated cellulosic, ceramic, or resin strips, especially against flies and mosquitos. For the control of fleas and ticks on livestock and domestic animals (pets), impregnated resin collars are used. A granular form of an impregnated resin strip is in use as an anthelmintic in domestic animals.

The various formulations include emulsifiable and oil-soluble concentrates, ready-for-use liquids, aerosols, granules, and impregnated strips. Formulations containing mixtures of dichlorvos with other insecticides, such as pyrethrins/piperonylbutoxide, tetramethrin, allethrins, chlorpyriphos, diazinon, propoxur, or fenitrothion, are also on the market.

3.2.3 Accidental release

Accidental spillages of dichlorvos could cause acute effects in water (e.g., mortality of aquatic species), but long-term effects are unlikely in view of its volatility and instability in humid environments.

4. ENVIRONMENTAL TRANSPORT, DISTRIBUTION, AND TRANSFORMATION

4.1 Transport and Distribution Between Media

Dichlorvos is not generally used for direct application on soil or to water. However, in intensive fish farming, dichlorvos is added directly to water. Any residues in soil resulting from the treatment of crops will be small and short-lived, due to volatilization and degradation. Therefore, contamination of ground water or surface water is unlikely to occur in normal practice. In air, dichlorvos is rapidly degraded, the rate depending on the humidity of the air.

4.2 Biotransformation

4.2.1 Abiotic degradation

In water, dichlorvos hydrolyses into dimethylphosphoric acid and DCA.

The photochemical degradation rate constant at environmentally important wavelengths (around 300 nm) was 265 x 10^{-7}/s at a concentration of 0.67 μg dichlorvos/cm^2 of glass plate, and the half-life was 7 h (Chen et al., 1984).

The relative persistence of dichlorvos on concrete, glass, and wood was investigated in the laboratory. The fastest loss occurred when it was applied to concrete; after 1 h, only 0.7% of the applied amount was present. This rapid loss was almost certainly due to alkaline decomposition. The disappearance rate on glass was less rapid, with a recovery of 1% dichlorvos 3 days after application. On wood, dichlorvos showed the greatest persistence; 65% and 39% of the applied dichlorvos still remained after one and 33 days, respectively (Hussey & Hughes, 1964).

When houses were treated for pest control with a total of 230-330 g dichlorvos as aerosol and 4 - 50 g as emulsion spray, the mean dichlorvos residue on the surface was 24 μg/100 cm^2 at the end of the first day, and fell to 6 μg/100 cm^2 by the end of 5 days (Das et al., 1983).

4.2.2 Biodegradation

Two ponds containing 9200 and 25 000 μg plankton/litre water, respectively, were treated with dichlorvos by spraying under the surface of the water. The initial dichlorvos concentration in the water was 325 μg/litre and the half-lives were 34 and 24 h, respectively (Grahl, 1979).

The biodegradation of dichlorvos in soil was tested in the laboratory using moist loam. The percentages of the applied amount (200 mg/kg soil) remaining in the soil after 1, 2, and 3 days were 93%,

62%, and 37%, respectively. Concentrations of free DCA in the soil were 9%, 7%, and 4%, respectively (Hussey & Hughes, 1964).

In studies on the fate of dichlorvos in soil, it was shown that *Bacillus cereus* grown on a nutrient medium containing 1000 mg dichlorvos/litre could use this compound as a sole carbon source but not as a sole phosphorus source. When soil columns were perfused with an aqueous solution containing 1000 mg dichlorvos/litre, the metabolic activity of *B. cereus* accounted for 30% of the loss of dichlorvos from the system over a 10-day period (Lamoreaux & Newland, 1978).

Dichlorvos in concentrations ranging from 0.1 to 100 mg/litre had little or no toxicity, as measured by the oxygen depletion caused by microorganisms degrading organic matter in sewage (Lieberman & Alexander, 1981, 1983).

Dichlorvos was converted to dichloroethanol, dichloroacetic acid, and ethyldichloroacetate by a microbial enrichment derived from sewage containing, principally, two species of *Pseudomonas* and one of *Bacillus*. The compounds were not formed in the absence of microbial cells. Inorganic phosphate was also generated in the presence of microorganisms, and dimethylphosphate was produced in the presence or absence of microbial cells (Lieberman & Alexander, 1981, 1983).

Pseudomonas melophthora, the bacterial symbiont of the apple maggot *(Rhagoletis pomonella)*,degraded dichlorvos mainly into water-soluble metabolites, using esterases (Boush & Matsumura, 1967). In addition, a strain of *Trichoderma viride,* a fungus isolated from soil, has the ability to degrade dichlorvos to water-soluble metabolites, probably through an oxidative pathway (Matsumura & Boush, 1968).

Dichlorvos is rapidly lost from leaf surfaces by volatilization and by hydrolysis, the half-life under laboratory conditions being of the order of a few hours. A small percentage of the dichlorvos deposited appears to penetrate into the waxy layers of plant tissues, where it persists longer and undergoes hydrolysis to DCA (FAO/WHO, 1968a, 1971a).

4.2.3 Bioaccumulation and biomagnification

Due to the transient nature of dichlorvos, no bioaccumulation or biomagnification occur in soil, water, plants, vertebrates, or invertebrates.

4.3 Ultimate Fate Following Use

Direct application of dichlorvos on crops or animals will result in residues disappearing rapidly by volatilization and hydrolysis. Airborne dichlorvos arising from fogging, spraying, or volatilization from impregnated strips is hydrolysed in the atmosphere to dimethylphosphate and DCA. Losses occur through ventilation and by absorption and hydrolysis on surfaces. Depending on the material, dichlorvos may be absorbed and diffuse into the material, or it may be hydrolysed on the surface.

5. ENVIRONMENTAL LEVELS AND HUMAN EXPOSURE

5.1 Environmental Levels

The occurrence of dichlorvos residues in the environment does not necessarily originate from the use of dichlorvos. It can also occur as a conversion product of trichlorphon (Miyamoto, 1959) and butonate (Dedek et al., 1979).

5.1.1 Air

Examples of indoor air concentrations resulting from the household and public health use of dichlorvos are given in Table 7. The air concentration varies according to the method of application (strips, spray cans, or fogging), the temperature, and humidity (Gillett et al., 1972). Using strips (one strip per 30 m^3), the concentration in the first week is in the range 0.1 - 0.3 mg/m^3, depending on the ventilation. During succeeding weeks, the concentration decreases to about 0.04 mg/m^3 and after 3 months to 0.01 mg/m^3 (Elgar & Steer, 1972).

5.1.2 Food

Data on residues in food commodities resulting from pre- or post-harvest treatment and from use on animals have been summarized by FAO/WHO (1967a, 1968a, 1971a, 1975a). Maximum residue limits, varying from 0.02 to 5 mg/kg, have been recommended for a range of commodities.

Frank et al. (1983) analysed 260 bovine and porcine fat samples collected in the period 1973-81 in Ontario. Only one sample contained a trace of dichlorvos.

Dichlorvos residues present in food commodities are readily destroyed during processing, e.g., washing, cooking. Hence, the chance that dichlorvos will occur in prepared meals is very low. This was confirmed by Abbott et al. (1970) in a total-diet study in the United Kingdom, in which no residues of dichlorvos were detected in the 462 sub-samples analysed.

In total-diet studies (including infant and toddler diets) carried out from 1964 to 1979 by the US Food and Drug Administration, no dichlorvos was found (Johnson et al., 1981a,b; Podrebarac, 1984).

Food samples, meals, and unwrapped ready-to-eat foodstuffs exposed under practical conditions to dichlorvos generated by resin strips showed mean residues of less than 0.05 mg/kg, with a range of < 0.01 - 0.1 mg/kg (Elgar et al., 1972a,b; Collins & de Vries, 1973). No residues of DCA (< 0.03 mg/kg; limit of detection) were detected in the ready-to-eat foodstuffs (Elgar et al., 1972b). Food and beverages exposed to experimental air concentrations of 0.04 - 0.58 mg/m^3 for 30 min contained dichlorvos residues of 0.005 - 0.5 mg/kg, with the

Table 7. Indoor air concentrations of dichlorvos following various applications

Location	Application	Dose[a]	Temperature (°C)	RH[b] (%)	Ventilation	Time after application	Concentration (mg/m^3)	Reference
food shops	resin strip	1 strip/ 30 m^3			normal	first week 4 weeks 10 weeks	0.03 0.02 0.01	Elgar et al. (1972b)
houses	resin strip	1 strip/ 30 m^3	18-35	20-60	normal	first week 2 - 3 weeks	0.06 - 0.17 0.01	Leary et al. (1974); Elgar & Steer (1972); Collins & de Vries (1973)
hospital wards	resin strip	1 strip/ 30 m^3	20-27	35-70	varied	several days 20 - 30 days	0.10 - 0.28 0.02	Cavagna et al. (1969)
hospital wards	strips of paper drenched in 50% dichlorvos solution hanging in the room for 24 - 36 h	0.2 ml ai/m^3	-	-	2 h	3 days	0.06	Schulze (1979)
		0.2 ml ai/m^3	17	-	2 h	66 h	0.1 - 0.3	
		0.2 ml ai/m^3	17		2 h	90 h	0.3	
		0.8 ml ai/m^3	30	high	2 h	3 h 46 h	3.7 0.6	

Table 7 (contd).

Location	Application	Dose[a]	Temperature (°C)	RH[b] (%)	Ventilation	Time after application	Concentration (mg/m^3)	Reference
houses	0.5% solution according to typical pest control practice	225 or 1200 ml	26	47-60	none	0 8 h 24 h	0.4 0.2 < 0.1	Neuwirth & White (1961)
bathroom (sealed)	0.5% solution wall spray	25 ml	26	60	none	0 4 h 24 h	1.1 0.3 < 0.1	Neuwirth & White (1961)
living room (experimental)	spray cans	2.3 mg ai/m^3	20-22		30 min 1 h	0 0	0.24 0.13	Sagner & Schöndube (1982)
	fogging	240 mg ai/m^3	20-22		none none 1 h 120 h	1 h 24 h 1 h 1 h	37 5.5 2.5 < 0.2	Sagner & Schöndube (1982)
appartments	0.5% solution	190 mg ai/m^2	26	82		0 - 2 h 2 - 24 h	0.5 0.2	Gold et al. (1984)

[a] ai = active ingredient.
[b] RH = relative humidity.

exception of margarine which contained up to 1.6 mg/kg (Dale et al., 1973).

5.2 General Population Exposure

Exposure of the general population to dichlorvos via air, water, or food, as a result of its agricultural or post-harvest use, is negligible. However, the household and public health use of dichlorvos is a source of exposure. The dichlorvos slow-release resin strip leads to exposure principally through inhalation from the air, but dermal absorption by contact with surfaces and oral ingestion of exposed food may also occur. Professional pest control with dichlorvos in buildings results in the same routes of exposure but to lower levels and for a shorter period (section 5.1).

Other sources of exposure are the use of household sprays and pet collars.

The increased use of organophosphorus insecticide on lawns and turf within parks and recreational areas presents a risk to human beings and animals. They may be potentially exposed to toxic levels of residues, although most product labels recommend that pets and children be kept off treated turf until the spray has dried. To safeguard against potential hazards, safe levels of dislodgeable residue have been estimated so that safe reentry intervals or reentry precautions can be established. In California, the estimated safe level of dislodgeable foliar dichlorvos residue is 0.06 $\mu g/cm^2$.

In studies carried out by Goh et al. (1986a,b), the dislodgeable foliar dichlorvos residue level immediately after application dropped rapidly during the first 2 - 6 h, and after 24 - 48 h, the residue was undetectable.

5.3 Occupational Exposure During Manufacture, Formulation, or Use

5.3.1 Air

Employees in a vaporizer production plant and adjoining packing rooms were exposed, on average, to 0.7 mg/m^3 air. The highest single value recorded was 3 mg/m^3 (Menz et al., 1974).

When air was analysed by Wright & Leidy (1980) in office and insecticide storage rooms in commercial pest control buildings and in vehicles, the concentrations of dichlorvos did not exceed 0.001 mg/m^3 air.

Gillenwater et al. (1971) measured maximum values of 2.4 - 7 mg/m^3 of dichlorvos in a large warehouse during weekly 6-h application periods. The amounts of dichlorvos dispersed per application ranged from 25 to 59 mg/m^3 and the average air concentration after 8 applications was 4 mg/m^3.

When the floors of a mushroom house were treated with a 10% solution of a 50% (w/v) dichlorvos emulsion (2 g dichlorvos/m^3 of house volume), air concentrations of dichlorvos were well below 1 mg/m^3. The air concentrations of DCA were approximately 1 mg/m^3, decreasing over 14 days to 0.3 mg/m^3 (Hussey & Hughes, 1964).

During thermal fogging by swingfog of 6 greenhouses (0.2 ml dichlorvos/m^3), the workplace concentration was 7 - 24 mg/m^3 (mean: 16 mg/m^3). Spraying of 12 glass and plastic green-houses resulted in workplace concentrations between 0.7 and 2.7 mg/m^3 (mean:1.3 mg/m^3). Field application by spraying resulted in air concentrations of 0.01 - 0.26 mg/m^3 (mean : 0.08 mg/m^3) (Wagner & Hoyer, 1975, 1976).

In a tobacco-drying unit used for mushroom production, dichlorvos was sprayed at 8 ml ai[a]/100 m^3, and the unit was kept closed for 24 h. Air concentrations decreased from 3.3 mg/m^3 to 0.006 mg/m^3 in 24 h. Treatment of the unit with paper strips drenched in 50% dichlorvos formulation (40 ml/100 m^3) resulted in air concentrations of 0.38 and 0.024 mg/m^3, 3 and 24 h, respectively, after treatment (Grübner, 1972).

Immediately after spraying plants in greenhouses with a 0.2 - 0.3% dichlorvos solution, the air concentration was 1.2 mg/m^3, decreasing to 0.01 mg/m^3 24 h later. When the plants were "shaken", air concentrations increased by 10 - 26% (Zotov et al., 1977).

The air levels of dichlorvos in a room of a residence were monitored during and after treatment with a pressurized home-fogger container. The study was performed to determine if the prescribed 30 min aeration period was sufficient to allow safe re-entry into a home or room. The air levels were below the industrial workplace permissible exposure level (PEL) of 1 mg/m^3, recommended by US OSHA, at the end of the aeration period. The dichlorvos dissipated quite slowly after that. Without ventilation, it took 18 h to reach an acceptable level. Because there is concern that infants and elderly or diseased persons occupying rooms almost 24 h/day, 7 days per week, might be more susceptible, the acceptable level for homes has been established at 1/40 of the PEL. Consequently, rooms treated with this type of application device and ventilated after treatment should not be re-entered for 10 h (Maddy et al., 1981a).

Dichlorvos is used to control Phorid flies in mushroom-growing houses. After its use in one of these houses in Ventura County in the USA in 1981, some workers complained of headaches and nausea upon re-entry after 30 min of ventilation. Monitoring of the mushroom houses, after the same treatment, revealed air concentrations of less than 0.1 mg/m^3 (0.01 ppm). Swab samples of exposed horizontal surfaces revealed a maximum of 0.026 μg/cm^2 (Maddy et al., 1981b).

---

[a] ai = active ingredient.

6. KINETICS AND METABOLISM

6.1 Absorption

Dichlorvos is readily absorbed via all routes of exposure. In the rat, dichlorvos taken orally is absorbed by the gastrointestinal tract, transported via the hepatic portal venous system to the liver, and detoxified before it reaches the systemic circulation (Gaines et al., 1966; Laws, 1966).

Air exhaled by anaesthetized and tracheotomized pigs exposed by inhalation to dichlorvos for up to 6 h revealed that, at dichlorvos concentrations of 0.1 - 2 mg/m³, the pigs retained 15 - 70% of the inhaled dichlorvos (Kirkland, 1971).

The percutaneous absorption of undiluted dichlorvos and solutions of dichlorvos applied (under a glass cover slip) to rabbit skin was calculated from the slope of the whole blood ChE activity inhibition curve. Water and acetone solutions did not increase absorption, whereas xylene and dimethylsulfoxide (DMSO) enhanced absorption (Shellenberger et al., 1965; Shellenberger, 1980). The results are summarized in Table 8.

Table 8. Effect of solvent on whole blood ChE activities and absorption rates[a] after percutaneous application of dichlorvos to rabbit skin

Solvent	ChE inhibition (%)	Time after application	Absorption (mg/min per cm²)
0.5 ml undiluted dichlorvos	30	2 h	3.8
+0.5 ml acetone	45	2 h	4.08
+0.5 ml water	45	2 h	4.29
+0.5 ml xylene	100	40 min	11.96
+0.5 ml DMSO	100	35 min	16.08

[a] Calculated from the slope of the enzyme inhibition curve.

6.1.1 Human studies

Dichlorvos was undetectable (less than 0.1 mg/litre) in the blood of two men immediately after exposure, one to air concentrations of 0.25 mg dichlorvos/m³ for 10 h and one to 0.7 mg dichlorvos/m³ for 20 h (Blair et al., 1975).

6.2 Distribution

6.2.1 Studies on experimental animals

6.2.1.1 Oral

^{32}P-Dichlorvos administered orally to rats at a single dose of 10 mg/kg body weight was found to be readily absorbed, distributed among the tissues, hydrolysed, and rapidly metabolized. Radioactivity was detected in the blood 15 min after administration, and the amount slowly decreased over subsequent days. The concentrations of ^{32}P in kidneys, liver, stomach, and intestines reached their maximum 1 h after dosing, and decreased within 1 day. The concentration in bone increased slowly with time due to the ^{32}P entering the inorganic phosphate pool of the organism. No sex differences were found (Casida et al., 1962).

When 1 mg of ^{14}C-methyldichlorvos was administered orally to rats, the gut, skin, and carcass contained 0.7%, 1.6%, and 5.2%, respectively, of the administered radioactivity, 4 days after dosing (Hutson & Hoadley, 1972b). In an earlier study on rats dosed orally with 1 mg vinyl-1-^{14}C-dichlorvos, the gut, skin, and carcass contained 1.7%, 7.5%, and 14%, respectively, of the ^{14}C, 4 days after dosing (Hutson et al., 1971a,b).

Twenty-four hours after the administration of a single oral dose of 0.2 mg vinyl-1-^{14}C-dichlorvos to mice, 26 - 34% of the radioactivity was found in the carcass (Hutson & Hoadley, 1972a). Syrian hamsters dosed with vinyl-1-^{14}C-dichlorvos retained similar percentages in the gut, skin, and carcass as did rats (Hutson & Hoadley, 1972a).

Fetuses from rabbits treated with daily oral doses of 5 mg dichlorvos/kg body weight for 25 days of gestation were found to contain no dichlorvos (Majewski et al., 1979).

In studies by Potter et al. (1973a), nine pigs received a single oral dose of vinyl-1-^{14}C-dichlorvos (approximately 40 mg dichlorvos/kg feed) formulated as slow-release PVC pellets. Sacrifices after 2, 7, and 14 days showed that all the tissues contained ^{14}C. The highest level of radioactivity, expressed as dichlorvos equivalent, was found in liver tissue after 2 days (33 mg/kg) and the lowest in brain tissue (2.5 mg/kg). In another study, pregnant sows were fed vinyl-1-^{14}C-dichlorvos or ^{36}Cl-dichlorvos in PVC pellets at 4 mg dichlorvos/kg body weight per day for the last third of the sow's gestation period. After farrowing, the sows and piglets, nursing from their own mothers, were kept for 21 days before being sacrificed. The tissues of the sows and piglets contained ^{14}C and ^{36}Cl residues ranging from 0.3 to 18 mg/kg tissue equivalents. In neither study, were residues of dichlorvos, DCA, desmethyldichlorvos, dichloroacetic acid, or dichloroethanol found in the tissues (Potter et al., 1973a,b).

No dichlorvos was found in muscle (fat) tissue of rabbits treated with daily oral doses of 5 mg dichlorvos/kg body weight for 2 weeks and sacrificed at intervals up to 48 h after the last dose (Majewski et al., 1979).

6.2.1.2 Inhalation

When groups of 3 rats and mice were exposed by inhalation to a concentration of 90 mg dichlorvos/m^3 air for 4 h, the rats exhibited mild signs of intoxication (lethargy, pupillary constriction). Concentrations of dichlorvos were very low or undetectable in blood (< 0.2 mg/kg), liver, testes, lung, and brain (< 0.1 mg/kg), while the kidneys and fat contained the highest concentrations (up to 2.4 and 0.4 mg/kg tissue, respectively). In rats, the values for the trachea were higher than those for the lungs, indicating perhaps that some dichlorvos is trapped in the trachea. When rats were exposed for 4 h to 10 mg/m^3 air, only the kidneys of the male animals contained measurable or detectable dichlorvos concentrations (0.08 mg/kg). Mice gave different results from rats, having higher concentrations of dichlorvos in fat, lung, and testes, and much lower concentrations in the kidneys. Exposure of male rats to 0.5 or 0.05 mg/m^3 for 14 days did not result in detectable residues (< 0.001 mg/kg) of dichlorvos in blood, liver, kidneys, renal fat, or lung tissue. However, in male rats exposed to approximately 50 mg dichlorvos/m^3, dichlorvos (1.7 mg/kg) was found in the kidneys after 2 and 4 h exposure time. On removal of the rats from the test atmosphere, the dichlorvos rapidly disappeared from the kidneys, with a half-life of 13.5 min. The rate of disappearance of dichlorvos in the blood was too rapid to measure; it could not be detected 15 min after exposure (Blair et al., 1975).

Short-term inhalation trials in anaesthesized pigs did not show the presence of intact dichlorvos or desmethyldichlorvos in blood or lung tissues. Even in the 2- to 4-h trials, the degradation proceeded to the stage where only methylphosphates and phosphoric acid could be detected (Loeffler et al., 1971). When young swine were exposed for 24 h to an atmosphere containing about 0.15 mg vinyl-1-^{14}C-dichlorvos/m^3, the ^{14}C content varied widely among the different tissues, but none contained dichlorvos (Loeffler et al., 1976).

6.2.1.3 Intraperitoneal

Nordgren et al. (1978) showed that within 1 min after a single intraperitoneal injection of 10 mg dichlorvos/kg body weight to mice, dichlorvos was detectable in the brain, but its concentration decreased within a few minutes.

Mice and rats treated repeatedly by intraperitoneal injection with 10 or 4 mg ^{32}P-dichlorvos/kg body weight showed hydrolysis products in the tissues within 2 h (Casida et al., 1962). When male rats were injected intraperitoneally with vinyl-1-^{14}C-dichlorvos, the mean 24-h retention percentages of administered radioactivity were: gut, 4%; skin, 7%; and carcass, 23% (Hutson et al., 1971b). No differences in the amount or distribution of radioactivity in the tissues of female rats given either a single oral or intraperitoneal dose of 4 mg vinyl-1-^{14}C-dichlorvos/kg body weight were reported (Casida et al., 1962).

6.2.1.4 Intravenous

The dichlorvos concentrations in the kidneys of three male rats, 10 and 30 min after a single intravenous injection, showed a considerable decrease, suggesting rapid metabolism of dichlorvos. As was the case after oral administration, dichlorvos could not be detected in the kidneys of female rats (Blair et al., 1975).

6.3 Metabolic Transformation

Early *in vitro* and *in vivo* studies indicated that detoxification of dichlorvos occurs in the liver (Casida et al., 1962; Hodgson & Casida, 1962; Gaines et al., 1966; Laws, 1966). *In vitro* studies have shown that rat liver degrades dichlorvos by two main enzymatic pathways, one being glutathione dependent and producing desmethyldichlorvos, and the other being glutathione independent and resulting in dimethylphosphate and DCA. The degradation of desmethyldichlorvos to DCA and monomethylphosphate was also found to be glutathione independent (Dicowsky & Morello, 1971). Sakai & Matsumura (1971) demonstrated the *in vitro* degradation of dichlorvos by human brain esterases.

Hodges & Casida (1962) have found that dichlorvos is hydrolysed by the soluble and mitochondrial fractions of the rat liver but not by the microsomes. DCA is reduced in the presence of NADH to dichloroethanol and possibly to dichloroacetate.

The rapidity of dichlorvos metabolism has been demonstrated in *in vitro* studies using fresh liver tissue. Ten minutes after mixing 1 mg dichlorvos with 1 g of liver tissue, 50% dichlorvos was recovered; after 123 min, only 0.4% remained (Majewski et al., 1979). However, it is not only liver tissue that metabolizes dichlorvos. ^{32}P-Dichlorvos was metabolized in the presence of blood and of adrenal, kidney, lung, and spleen tissues, mainly to dimethylphosphate. Desmethyldichlorvos, monomethylphosphate, and inorganic phosphate were also found (Hodgson & Casida, 1962; Loeffler et al., 1971).

The identification of dichlorvos metabolites has been undertaken in *in vivo* studies of mice (Casida et al., 1962; Hutson & Hoadley, 1972a,b), rats (Casida et al., 1962; Bull & Ridgeway, 1969; Hutson et al., 1971b; Hutson & Hoadley, 1972b), Syrian hamsters (Hutson & Hoadley, 1972a), pigs (Loeffler et al., 1971, 1976; Page et al., 1972; Potter et al., 1973a,b), goats (Casida et al., 1962), cows (Casida et al., 1962), and human beings (Hutson & Hoadley, 1972a), after different routes of administration using radiolabelled dichlorvos. In general, the metabolism of dichlorvos in the various species is similar and rapid. Differences between species are related to the rate of metabolite formation rather than to the nature of the metabolites.

In the mouse, *O*-desmethylation is a more important route of dichlorvos detoxification than it is in the rat (Table 9), as indicated by the larger amounts of radioactivity excreted in the mice as desmethyldichlorvos.

Table 9. Isotope dilution analysis of urine from mammals treated orally with vinyl-1-^{14}C-dichlorvos[a]

Metabolite measured	Proportion of administered radioactivity as urinary metabolite (%)			
	rat	mouse	hamster	man
hippuric acid	1.7	0.6	1.0	0.4
desmethyldichlorvos	2.2	18.5	-[b]	0.15
urea (isolated as the nitrate salt)	0.6	0.6	-[b]	0.1

[a] From: Hutson & Hoadley (1972a).
[b] Not measured.

Desmethyldichlorvos arises from the hydrolysis of the methyl oxygen-phosphate bond and is further degraded into DCA, monomethylphosphate, and dimethylphosphate (Casida et al., 1962; Hodgson & Casida, 1962; Bradway et al., 1977). *S*-methyl-glutathione is formed along with desmethyldichlorvos, and is degraded to methylmercapturic acid and excreted in the urine (Hutson & Hoadley, 1972b).

The two major routes of metabolism of the vinyl portion of the dichlorvos molecule lead to: (a) dichloroethanol glucuronide, and (b) hippuric acid, urea, carbon dioxide, and other endogenous biochemicals which give rise to high levels of radioactivity in the tissues for a few days after dosing with vinyl-1-^{14}C-dichlorvos. Both pathways have been shown to occur in man, owing to the presence of these compounds in the urine (Hutson & Hoadley, 1972a). In laboratory animals most of the observed radioactivity in carcasses and tissues was present as glycine, serine, and other normal body components, indicating that the vinyl carbon atoms of dichlorvos enter the 2-carbon metabolic pool (Hutson et al., 1971b; Page et al., 1971; Hutson & Hoadley, 1972b; Loeffler et al., 1976). No evidence of accumulation of dichlorvos or potentially toxic metabolites was found. A scheme of the metabolites of dichlorvos in mammals is given in Fig. 1.

6.3.1 Metabolites

When ^{32}P-dimethylphosphate (500 mg/kg body weight) was administered orally to a male rat almost the entire dose was eliminated. The urine contained about 50% unmetabolized

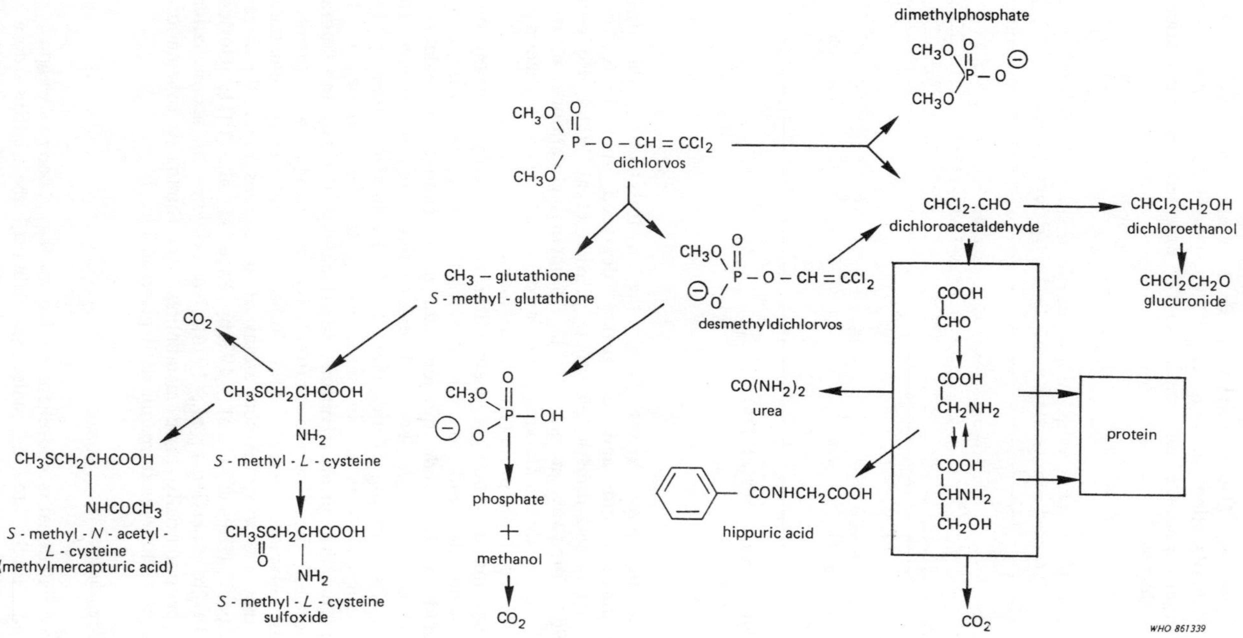

Fig. 1. Metabolism of dichlorvos in mammals.

dimethylphosphate. On the other hand, a rat orally dosed with ^{32}P-desmethyldichlorvos (500 mg/kg body weight) eliminated about 14% of the dose via urine in 90 h, 86% of the radioactivity being phosphoric acid and 14% unchanged desmethyldichlorvos. The very high proportion of radioactivity in the bone was indicative of rapid degradation to phosphoric acid (Casida et al., 1962).

Following the intraperitoneal injection of 1-^{14}C-DCA or 1-^{14}C-dichloroethanol to female rats, 32% of the radioactivity was expired as carbon dioxide within 24 h (Casida et al., 1962).

6.4 Elimination and Excretion in Expired Air, Faeces, and Urine

6.4.1 Human studies

Eight hours after a human male consumed 5 mg of vinyl-1-^{14}C-dichlorvos in orange juice, 27% of the radioactivity had been eliminated as ^{14}C-carbon dioxide. Approximately 8% had been excreted by the urine within one day following dosing. Urinary excretion of radioactivity decreased gradually and by day 9 none was detectable (Hutson & Hoadley, 1972a).

The concentration of dimethylphosphate in the urine of three pesticide control operators spraying houses with dichlorvos ranged from 0.32 to 1.4 μg at the end of the day's work (Das et al., 1983).

6.4.2 Studies on experimental animals

6.4.2.1 Oral

Dosing rats orally with ^{32}P-dichlorvos (0.1 - 80 mg/kg body weight) resulted in a recovery of 60 - 70% of the administered radioactivity in the urine and approximately 10% in the faeces over a 6-day period following dosing (Casida et al., 1962).

After the oral administration of methyl-^{14}C-dichlorvos to rats (1 mg) and mice (0.5 mg), the excretion of radioactivity was rapid. The major route of elimination after 4 days was the urine (approximately 60%), followed by expired air (approximately 16%) (Hutson & Hoadley, 1972b).

Rats given an oral dose of vinyl-1-^{14}C-dichlorvos (1 mg per animal) eliminated 10 - 20% of the ^{14}C in the urine, 3 - 5% in the faeces, and approximately 40% as expired carbon dioxide over 4 days following dosing (Hutson et al., 1971a,b).

A comparison between the excretion by rat, mouse, hamster, and man 24 h after oral dosing with vinyl-1-^{14}C-dichlorvos is given in Table 10 (Hutson & Hoadley, 1972a).

A cow treated orally with 20 mg/kg body weight ^{32}P-dichlorvos eliminated 40% of the radioactivity in the urine and 50% in the faeces. In the milk, the level of organosoluble radioactivity was significantly above background only within the first 2 h (Casida et al., 1962).

Table 10. Comparison of percentages of radioactivity excreted by males 24 h after oral ingestion of vinyl-1-^{14}C-dichlorvos[a]

Excretion route	Rat (3)	Mouse (1)	Hamster (2)	Man (1)
urine	9.8	27.4	14.7	7.6
faeces	1.5	3.2	2.9	-
carbon dioxide	28.8	23.1	33.5	27 (8 h only)

[a] Number of animals are given in parentheses.

6.4.2.2 Parenteral

The elimination of a single intraperitoneal injection of vinyl-1-^{14}C-dichlorvos (4 mg/kg body weight) from female rats was similar to the elimination after oral dosing. A goat treated subcutaneously with 1.5 mg ^{32}P-dichlorvos/kg body weight excreted 79% of the radioactivity in the urine and 11% in the faeces. Two cows received an intravenous or a subcutaneous injection with 1 mg ^{32}P-dichlorvos/kg body weight. Of the radioactivity which was recovered, 70 - 80% was in the urine and approximately 14% in the faeces (Casida et al., 1962).

6.5 Retention and Turnover

6.5.1 Biological half-life

In studies by Blair et al. (1975), the metabolism of dichlorvos was found to be so rapid that the biological half-life in blood could not be determined. No intact dichlorvos could be demonstrated in the blood or tissues of animals exposed by routes other than parenteral injection. Only after exposure for 4 h to an atmospheric concentration of 90 mg dichlorvos/m^3 could dichlorvos be detected in most tissues of the rat and mouse. Following exposure at 50 mg/m^3, for 2 or 4 h, the half-life in the rat kidney was 13.5 min.

The intraperitoneal injection of 10 mg dichlorvos/kg body weight into mice increased the accumulation of ACh in the brain and caused an inhibition of ChE activity. Symptoms of toxicity were clearly recognizable after 15 min, and they disappeared almost completely after 60 min. The ChE activity and ACh levels reached their minimum and maximum, respectively, at 15 min. The maximum concentration of dichlorvos in the brain was reached after 1 min and decreased thereafter, rapidly reaching the baseline level after 3 min (Nordgren et al., 1978).

6.5.2 *Body burden*

There is no evidence for the storage of dichlorvos or its metabolites in the tissues of animals. Small fractions of the carbon, phosphorus, and chlorine derived from dichlorvos are retained in the body for several days because their turnover rate is the same as that for identical materials from other origins.

6.5.3 *Indicator media*

The determination of dichloroethanol in urine as a means of monitoring the exposure of human beings to dichlorvos is not sufficiently sensitive to detect levels arising from vapour exposure through normal use. However, it could serve as the basis for a specific detection method for the accidental ingestion of high levels (Hutson & Hoadley, 1972a). Two other methods can be used: (a) determination of the blood ChE activity; or (b) determination of dimethylphosphate in urine by a rather complicated method (Blair & Roderick, 1976). Neither method is specific when exposure to other organophosphate or carbamate compounds, or to compounds that also metabolize to dimethylphosphate, may have occurred.

7. EFFECTS ON ORGANISMS IN THE ENVIRONMENT

7.1 Microorganisms

Lal (1982) reviewed the accumulation, metabolism, and effects of organophosphorus insecticides on microorganisms.

Microorganisms undoubtedly have the ability to metabolize organophosphorus insecticides; however, there are still large gaps in our knowledge. It also seems clear that chemical, photochemical, physical, and biological factors may influence the metabolism of dichlorvos by microorganisms.

7.1.1 Algae and plankton

The dose of dichlorvos producing 50% growth inhibition of the unicellular alga *Euglena gracilis* has been quoted as 3.5 mg/litre (Butler, 1977).

Treating eutrophic carp ponds with 0.325 mg/litre killed *Cladocera* (predominantly *Bosmina* and *Daphnia* species) and decreased *Copepoda* (mainly *Cyclops*). This was offset by increased development of *Rotatoria* (mainly *Polyarthra* and *Brachionus* species) and phytoplankton (mainly *Scenedesmus* and *Pediastrum* species), so that the total plankton biomass changed only slightly (Grahl et al., 1981).

7.1.2. Fungi

Dichlorvos (in the range 10 - 80 mg/litre) has been found to affect citric acid fermentation in *Aspergillus niger* grown in an artificial medium. Inhibition of the fermentation was marked only at 40 and 80 mg/litre (Rahmatullah et al., 1978; Ali et al., 1979c). It appears from the decreased uptake of inorganic phosphorus that dichlorvos may have an interfering action on oxidative metabolism in *A. niger*. The potential for inhibiting citrinin production by *Penicillium citrinum* was investigated. Dichlorvos inhibited citrinin production by 76% at 100 μg/litre and by 48% at 10 μg/litre (Draughon & Ayres, 1978). The effect of dichlorvos on the survival time and the membrane potential of the slime mould *Physarum polycephalum* was studied in a laboratory test system. The threshold value for both these effects was found to be 300 mg/litre for technical dichlorvos and 30 mg/litre for the pure chemical (Terayama et al., 1978).

The influence of dichlorvos on 17 soil fungi, cultivated in artificial medium, was tested. Dose levels of 0, 10, 30, 60, and 120 mg/kg were used during a test period of 21 days, and the effect on the growth and morphology of the fungi was studied. In general, a growth depression was found, but its extent depended on the fungal strain. Occasionally growth was either unaffected or even stimulated (Jakubowska & Nowak, 1973).

7.1.3. Bacteria

Dichlorvos has been found not to influence the overall metabolic processes of *Escherichia coli* and *Enterobacter aerogenes* at doses up to 250 mg/litre (Grahl et al., 1980) and was not toxic for a sewage isolate at up to 10 mg/litre (Rosenberg et al., 1979). In poultry effluent slurry, concentrations of 100 and 1000 mg/litre did not significantly reduce coliform populations, but 10 000 mg/litre caused almost complete death. Therefore, residues of dichlorvos used for fly control in layer houses can significantly reduce the enteric coliform populations that are essential to the conversion of organic nitrogen to inorganic nitrogen in poultry waste effluent (Ballington et al., 1978).

In studies by Lieberman & Alexander (1981), dichlorvos (0.1 - 100 mg/litre) had little or no toxicity for microorganisms degrading organic matter in sewage, as measured by respiratory activity, degradation, and nitrification.

Incubation of dichlorvos with inocula of ruminal bacteria or ciliated protozoa under anaerobic conditions suggests that dichlorvos is not utilized by the organisms for growth, nor does it stimulate endogenous gas production. However, it does, in certain instances, affect volatile fatty acid production (Williams, 1977).

The growth of *Bacillus thuringiens* var *th.* was not inhibited by dichlorvos (Dougherty et al., 1971).

7.2 Aquatic Organisms

Reviews of the acute and chronic effects of pesticides on aquatic organisms have been made by Brungs et al. (1977), Livingston (1977), and Kenaga (1979).

The toxicity of a chemical for aquatic organisms is influenced by many factors such as the stage of development of the organism and the composition, pH, oxygen content, and hardness of the water. In this short review, these factors are not discussed in detail.

7.2.1 Fish

7.2.1.1 Acute toxicity

The acute toxicity of dichlorvos for both freshwater and estuarine species of fish is moderate to high. The available data are summarized in Table 11.

Variations in water hardness from 44 to 162 mg/litre and in pH from 6 to 9 did not alter the toxicity of dichlorvos for cutthroat or lake trout (Johnson & Finley, 1980).

Table 11. Acute toxicity of dichlorvos for fish

Species	Mass or length	Temperature (°C)	96-h LC_{50} (mg/litre)	Reference
<u>Freshwater</u>				
Clarias batrachus	26 - 31 g	-	8.9	Verma et al. (1983)
Carp *(Cyprinus carpio)*	8 mm 6 g	20 - 23 23	0.34 20[a]	Verma et al. (1981d) Yamane et al. (1974)
Mosquito fish *(Gambusia affinis)*	0.2 g	17	5.3	Johnson & Finley (1980)
Blue gill *(Lepomis macrochirus)*	1.5 g	18	0.9	Johnson & Finley (1980)
African catfish *(Mystus vittatus)*	6 - 10 g	18	0.5	Verma et al. (1980, 1981a)
Ophiopcephalus punctatus	40 - 55 g	18	2.3	Verma et al. (1981a)
Fathead minnow *(Pimephales promelas)*	0.7 g	17	12	Johnson & Finley (1980)
Harlequin fish *(Rasbora heteromorpha)*	-	20	7.8[b]	Alabaster (1969)
Singii *(Saccobranchus fossilis)*	5 - 10 g	18	6.6	Verma et al. (1982a)
Cutthroat trout *(Salmo clarki)*	2.5 g	12	0.2	Johnson & Finley (1980)

Table 11 (contd).

Lake trout (*Salvelinus namaycush*)	0.3 g	12	0.2	Johnson & Finley (1980)
Tilapia mossambica	3 - 10 cm	29	1.4 - 1.9	Rath & Misra (1979a)
<u>Estuarine</u>				
American eel (*Anguilla rostrata*)	0.14 g	20	1.8	Eisler (1970)
Mummichog (*Fundulus heteroclitus*)	1.7 g	20	2.7	Eisler (1970)
Striped killifish (*Fundulus majalis*)	0.92 g	20	2.3	Eisler (1970)
Atlantic silverside (*Menidia menidia*)	0.8 g	20	1.3	Eisler (1970)
Striped mullet (*Mugil cephalus*)	1 - 6 g	20	0.23	Eisler (1970)
Northern puffer (*Sphaeroidus maculatus*)	100 g	20	2.3	Eisler (1970)
Bluehead (*Thalassoma bifasciatum*)	5.4 g	20	1.4	Eisler (1970)

a 24-h LC_{50}.
b 48-h LC_{50}.

In studies by Yamane et al. (1974), young carp were exposed to a concentration of 25 mg dichlorvos/litre water for 45 min. The ChE activity (histochemically determined) of many tissues, including the stratum griseum periventriculare, sarcolemma, and liver, was inhibited or totally lost.

7.2.1.2 Short-term toxicity

Sublethal concentrations of dichlorvos (0.5 - 1 mg/litre) have been found to decrease the respiratory rates of *Tilapia mossambica* (3 different age groups) exposed for up to 3 weeks. When the exposed fish were transferred to fresh water, the rate did not completely return to its pre-exposure value (Rath & Misra, 1979b). Liver and brain ChE activity showed considerable inhibition when a group of *T. mossambica* was exposed to dichlorvos (0.25 - 1.25 mg/litre water) for periods of up to 4 weeks. At 7-day intervals, fish were studied or transferred to clean water. The degree of enzyme inhibition was related to the dichlorvos concentration and length of exposure. In all age groups of fish, brain tissue exhibited a higher degree of ChE inhibition than liver. Small fish were more susceptible to dichlorvos with respect to AChE activity. When the fish were transferred to clean water, most of the fish recovered their AChE activity, the recovery being greater in liver than in brain. Small fish exhibited a comparatively high level of recovery. The degree of recovery was inversely related to the length of exposure (Rath & Misra, 1981).

Melanin dispersion in *T. mossambica* exposed to 1 mg/litre water for 15 days was stimulated indirectly by the inhibition of ChE activity. The original colour was regained within 96 h after transfer of the fish to clean water (Rath & Misra, 1980).

Exposure of *Mystus vittatus* (collected in the environment) to sublethal concentrations of dichlorvos (0.045 or 0.09 mg/litre) for 30 days caused dose-related increases in serum glutamic-oxaloacetic and glutamic-pyruvic transaminase levels (Verma et al., 1981b), increases in alkaline phosphatase, acid phosphatase, and glucose-6-phosphatase levels in serum (Verma et al., 1984), decreases in the levels of these enzymes in liver, kidneys, and gills (Verma et al., 1981c), an increase in glucose levels in blood, and a decrease in liver glycogen. Blood lactate and muscle glycogen were unaffected (Verma et al., 1983). At 0.09 mg/litre, blood clotting time, mean corpuscular haemoglobin and mean corpuscular haemoglobin concentration decreased, and the number of leukocytes increased. Other haematological parameters did not show any abnormalities (Verma et al., 1982b). From these results, a no-observed-adverse-effect concentration of 0.03 mg/litre was derived.

In studies by Verma & Tonk (1984), *Heteropneustes (Saccobranchus) fossilis* was exposed to dichlorvos for 30 days at a concentration of 0.44 mg/litre. Respiration, haematological parameters, and the activities of two enzymes (one of them AChE) in liver, kidneys, and gills were determined. The respiration rate decreased, and blood concentrations of sodium and chloride ions and glucose increased significantly, whereas the cholesterol level and clotting time were decreased. A significant reduction in the AChE activity of the three tissues was found.

Vadhva & Hasan (1986) studied the effect of dichlorvos (at 0, 3, 6, and 9 mg/litre water) on various lipid fractions and lipid peroxidation in the central nervous system of *Heteropneustes fossilis*. After one week's exposure, the results indicated that dichlorvos caused dose-related increases in total lipids, cholesterol-esterified fatty acid, and lipid peroxidation in various regions of the brain and spinal cord but a consistent decrease in the level of phospholipids in these regions of the central nervous system.

Exposure of *Clarias batrachus* to 0.5 - 2.2 mg dichlorvos/litre and *Saccobranchus fossilis* to 0.4 - 1.6 mg/litre for 30 days was found to increase blood glucose and decrease liver glycogen, whereas blood lactate and muscle glycogen were normal (Verma et al., 1983).

The estimated "maximum acceptable toxicant concentration" (MATC)[a] for the larvae of *Cyprinus carpio* was 0.016 - 0.020 mg/litre based on a 60-day study (Verma et al., 1981d).

7.2.2 Invertebrates

The acute toxicity of dichlorvos for aquatic insects and crustaceans is extremely high (Table 12). As might be expected from an organophosphorus insecticide, aquatic invertebrates are about three orders of magnitude more susceptible to dichlorvos than are fish, and freshwater crustaceans are particularly sensitive.

A study was carried out to determine the influence of a number of pesticides on the "hatchability" of *Artemia salina* dry eggs. No effect was found at 10 mg dichlorvos/litre in the aqueous system (Kuwabara et al., 1980).

When prawns *(Macrobrachium lamarrei)* were exposed to dichlorvos at concentrations of 0.31 or 0.62 mg/litre for 96 h, a decrease in hepatic glycogen and an increase in the blood glucose level were found (Omkar & Shukla, 1984). Possibly, the phosphorylase activity of the hepatopancreas and muscle increased due to the inhibition of AChE activity and the consequent accumulation of acetylcholine at neurosynaptic junctions. The latter resulted in an induction of the secretion of the sinus gland, which enhanced glycogenolysis.

7.3 Terrestrial Organisms

7.3.1 Birds

7.3.1.1 Acute oral toxicity

Dichlorvos has a high oral toxicity for birds (Table 13). The signs of intoxication are typical of organophosphorus poisoning, namely

---

[a] Maximum concentration at which no effect was seen.

Table 12. Acute toxicity of dichlorvos for non-target aquatic insects and Crustacea

Species	Temperature (°C)	48-h LC_{50} (µg/litre)	96-h LC_{50} (µg/litre)	Reference
Insects (stone flies)				
Pteronarcys californica	15	-	0.1	Johnson & Finley (1980)
Crustacea (fresh water)				
Water flea (*Daphnia pulex*)	15	0.07	-	Johnson & Finley (1980)
Water flea (*Simocephalus serrulatus*)	21	0.28	-	Johnson & Finley (1980)
Amphipod (*Gammarus lacustris*)	21	-	0.5	Johnson & Finley (1980)
Crustacea (estuarine)				
Sand shrimp (*Crangon septemspinosa*)	-	12	4	Eisler (1969)
Grass shrimp (*Palaemonetes vulgaris*)	-	300	15	Eisler (1969)
Hermit crab (*Pagurus longicarpus*)	-	52	45	Eisler (1969)

Table 13. Acute oral LD_{50} values for birds

Species	Age	Vehicle	LD_{50} (mg/kg body weight)	Reference
Red-winged blackbird *(Agelaius phoenicius)* (male)		propylene glycol	13.3	Schafer & Brunton (1979)
Mallard duck *(Anas platyrhynchos)* (male)	5 - 7 months	capsule	7.8	Tucker & Crabtree (1970)
Common pigeon *(Columba livia)*		propylene glycol	24	Schafer & Brunton (1979)
Quail[a] *(Coturnix coturnix)* (female)		propylene glycol	24	Schafer & Brunton (1979)
Domestic fowl *(Gallus domesticus)* (male)	21 days	aqueous suspension	6.5	Naidu et al. (1978)
	6 - 8 months	aqueous suspension	30	Dmitriev & Kozhemyakin (1975)
House sparrow *(Passer domesticus)*		propylene glycol	17.8	Schafer & Brunton (1979)
Ring-necked pheasant *(Phasianus colchicus)* (male)	3 months	capsule	11	Tucker & Crabtree (1970)
Common grackle *(Quiscalus quiscula)*		propylene glycol	13.3	Schafer & Brunton (1979)
Starling *(Sturnus vulgaris)*	adult	propylene glycol	12	Schafer (1972)
	-	propylene glycol	42.1	Schafer & Brunton (1979)

[a] Hattori et al. (1974) carried out studies on Japanese quail and found LD_{50} values of 22 and 26 respectively, for male and female (no details available).

salivation, lachrymation, tremors, and terminal convulsions. They usually appear shortly after dosing, and, at lethal doses, death occurs within 1 h. Survivors appear to recover completely 24 h after dosing. Various internal haemorrhages were found at autopsy in sacrificed survivors of treated pheasants and Mallard ducks (Tucker & Crabtree, 1970).

7.3.1.2 Short-term toxicity

In short-term dietary studies, dichlorvos has been found to be slightly to moderately toxic for birds (Table 14).

In the study with 7-day-old male chicks, there was weight loss and 50% mortality at 500 mg/kg diet. Marked, dose-related inhibition of brain ChE activity occurred at 50, 100, and 500 mg/kg diet, but no effects were noted at a level of 10 mg/kg diet (Naidu et al., 1978).

Canaries, Indian finches, and budgerigars, continuously exposed to dichlorvos vapour (0.14 mg/m^3) for 5 days, did not show any overt signs of intoxication, but a reduction in ChE levels in plasma and brain was observed in canaries and Indian finches (Brown et al., 1968).

7.3.1.3 Field experience

Caution has been advised in the use and handling of dichlorvos where birds might be exposed (Whitehead, 1971). The necessity for this warning can be illustrated by the following cases. Adult mallards feeding near horse mangers containing dichlorvos-treated feed were found dead within a short time. At necropsy, excessive amounts of mucus covering the mucosa of the proventriculus and scattered petechiae along medial edges of liver lobes were observed. The small and large intestines were markedly extended, and crystals were noted in the gizzard. Brain ChE activity was inhibited by 75 - 80% (Ludke & Locke, 1976). Domestic fowl, which had accidental access to the faeces of a horse dosed with dichlorvos pellets, picked out the pellets and more than 30 birds died during the next 24 h (Lloyd, 1973). A mass poisoning occurred in chickens following consumption of accidentally contaminated drinking-water (Egyed & Bendheim, 1977). English game bantams died after consuming wheat contaminated with 300 mg dichlorvos/kg wheat (Reece, 1982).

*7.3.2 **Invertebrates***

Dichlorvos was toxic for silkworm larvae when for 4 h they were fed mulberry leaves previously sprayed with dilute dichlorvos emulsions. Spray concentrations giving 50% mortality ranged from 1.56 to 6.25 mg/litre (Aratake & Kayamura, 1973).

No adverse effects were observed on the hatchability and general condition of first instar silkworm larvae hatched in the following generation when 5th instar larvae were fed mulberry leaves pre-treated with 3 mg dichlorvos/kg of leaf (Yamanoi, 1980).

Table 14. Dietary LD_{50} values for birds

Species	Age (days)	Duration of feeding (days)	LD_{50} (mg/kg diet)	Reference
Mallard duck *(Anas platyrhynchos)*	16	8[a]	5000	Hill et al. (1975)
	5	8[a]	1310	Hill et al. (1975)
Japanese quail *(Coturnix japonica)*	14	8[a]	300	Hill et al. (1975)
Domestic fowl *(Gallus domesticus)* (male)	7	28	500	Naidu et al. (1978)
Ring-necked pheasant *(Phasianus colchicus)*	10	8[a]	570	Hill et al. (1975)

[a] The median lethal dietary dose (LD_{50}) during an 8-day test including 5 days of treated diet followed by 3 days of untreated diet.

7.3.3 *Honey bees*

Dichlorvos is highly toxic for honey bees. Atkins et al. (1973) found in laboratory studies an LD_{50} of 0.495 μg/bee in 48 h (topical application of dust; 26.7 °C; relative humidity 65%). Beran (1979) obtained an oral LD_{50} of 0.29 μg/g body weight and an LD_{50} (topical application) value of 0.65 μg/g body weight. This high toxicity has led dichlorvos to be classified in the most toxic category for bees in Austria and the USA.

When honeycombs were exposed to dichlorvos vapour from dichlorvos resin strips for 4 months, the combs absorbed the insecticide and were toxic to bees for approximately one month after exposure ceased. Contamination of the bees appeared to be by fumigant rather than contact action (Clinch, 1970).

7.3.4 *Miscellaneous*

Dichlorvos was highly toxic for the predatory mite *Amblyseius longispinosus* in contact trials. Residual toxicity disappeared within 6 days, the susceptibility being the same as that of *Phytoseiulus persimilis* (Shinkaji & Adachi, 1978).

8. EFFECTS ON EXPERIMENTAL ANIMALS AND *IN VITRO* TEST SYSTEMS

A more complete treatise on the effects of organophosphorus insecticides in general, especially their short- and long-term effects on the nervous system, will be found in Environmental Health Criteria 63: Organophosphorus Insecticides - A General Introduction (WHO, 1986).

8.1 Single Exposures

Dichlorvos is moderately to highly toxic when administered in single doses by various routes to a variety of animal species (Table 15). It is less toxic via the dermal and oral routes than by parenteral routes. The signs of intoxication by all exposure routes are typical of organophosphorus poisoning, i.e., salivation, lacrimation, diarrhoea, tremors, and terminal convulsions, with death occurring from respiratory failure. In addition, lethargy, ataxia, hypersensitivity to noise, splayed gait, and paresis may be observed. The signs are usually apparent shortly after dosing and, at lethal doses, death occurs within 1 h. Survivors appear to recover completely 24 h after dosing.

The acute inhalational LC_{50} values for mice and rats are summarized in Table 16. The apparent differences in the LC_{50}s may be the result of the type of exposure of the animal (whole body or head only), whether the studies were carried out with dichlorvos vapour or atomized particles of spray (with or without vehicle), or differences in the purity of the dichlorvos. Moreover, since dichlorvos adheres strongly to surfaces including glass, the out-going air has a significantly lower concentration of dichlorvos than the air coming into the chamber, if the system is not yet equilibrated.

No macroscopic abnormalities were observed in mice or rats 2 weeks after a single exposure (MacDonald, 1982).

8.1.1 Domestic animals

When cattle and sheep were treated orally with a single dose of dichlorvos, 10 mg/kg body weight was toxic for calves and 25 mg/kg body weight for sheep. For the latter a dose of 10 mg/kg body weight was without effects (Radeleff & Woodard, 1957).

8.1.2 Potentiation

Potentiation studies on male rats indicated that oral administration of dichlorvos with 22 other organophosphate pesticides resulted in no (or very little) potentiation, while administration with malathion showed a marked potentiation (Narcisse, 1967; Kimmerle & Lorke, 1968). However, Cohen & Ehrich (1976) found that the anti-ChE action of 800 mg malathion/kg body weight (injected intraperitoneally)

Table 15. The acute toxicity (LD_{50}) of dichlorvos for experimental animals

Species	Route	Purity	Vehicle	LD_{50} (mg/kg)	Reference
Mouse (male)	oral	unknown	Eryfor EL or other solvents	68 - 90	Vrbovsky et al. (1959); Ueda et al. (1960)
Mouse	oral	80%	unknown	87	Sasinovich (1968, 1970)
Mouse	oral	97%	aqueous polysorbate 80	133 - 139[a]	Haley et al. (1975)
Mouse (male)	oral	98%	corn oil	140	Isshiki et al. (1983)
Mouse	oral	unknown	aqueous	124 - 275[a]	Yamashita (1960, 1962); Holmstedt et al. (1978)
Mouse (male)	subcutaneous	unknown	propylene glycol and other solvents	13 - 33	Ueda et al. (1960); Jaques (1964)
Mouse	subcutaneous	unknown	aqueous	20 - 26	Yamashita (1960, 1962); Holmstedt et al. (1978)
Mouse (male)	dermal	unknown	different solvents	206 & 395[b]	Ueda et al. (1960)
Mouse	intraperitoneal	technical	corn oil	28	Vrbovsky et al. (1959); Casida et al. (1962)

Table 15 (contd).

Mouse	intraperitoneal	unknown	aqueous	28 - 41[a]	Holmstedt et al. (1978)
Mouse	intravenous	unknown	aqueous	8 - 10	Holmstedt et al. (1978)
Rat	oral	90 - 99%	peanut oil and other solvents	56 - 96[a]	Durham et al. (1957); Narcisse (1967); Gaines (1969)
Rat (male)	oral	unknown	Eryfor EL and other solvents	46 - 110	Vrbovsky et al. (1959); Ueda et al. (1960)
Rat	oral	80%	unknown	65	Sasinovich (1968, 1970)
Rat	oral	unknown	aqueous	30	Holmstedt et al. (1978)
Rat	dermal	unknown	xylene	75 - 107[a]	Durham et al. (1957); Gaines (1969)
Rat	dermal	80%	unknown	113	Sasinovich (1968, 1970)
Rat	subcutaneous	95%	dimethylsulfoxide	72	Brown & Stevenson (1962)
Rat (male)	intraperitoneal	unknown	Eryfor EL	18	Vrbovsky et al. (1959)

Table 15 (contd).

Species	Route	Purity	Vehicle	LD_{50} (mg/kg)	Reference
Guinea-pig	subcutaneous	95%	undiluted	28	Brown & Stevenson (1962)
Syrian hamster	intraperitoneal	-	suspension in water	30	Dzwonkowska & Hübner (1986)
Rabbit	oral	93%	unknown	12.5	Desi et al. (1978)
Rabbit	oral	80%	unknown	22.5	Sasinovich (1968, 1970)
Rabbit	dermal	80%	unknown	205	Sasinovich (1968, 1970)
Cat	oral	80%	unknown	28	Sasinovich (1968, 1970)
Dog	oral		in capsule	100 - 316	Kodama (1960)
Swine (40- to 60-day-old)	oral	technical	in capsule	157	Stanton et al. (1979)
Domestic fowl (chicken)	oral	technical	in capsule	15	Sherman & Ross (1961)

a The LD_{50}s are often slightly different in males and females. Furthermore, it is clear that the purity of the dichlorvos tested and the vehicle used has an influence on the toxicity.

b The two values were obtained using two different solvents.

Table 16. Inhalational LC_{50} values for dichlorvos

Species	Purity	Type of exposure	Duration	LC_{50} (mg/m^3)	Reference
Mouse	80%	vapour whole body	4 h	13	Sasinovich (1968, 1970)
Mouse	98%	vapour head only	4 h	> 218	MacDonald (1982)
Mouse (male)	unknown; in solvent C[a]	vapour whole body	4 h	310	Ueda et al. (1960)
Rat (male)	unknown	unknown, but uptake by inhalation only	1 h	455	Kimmerle & Lorke (1968)
Rat (male)	84.1% polyethylene glycol	whole body	1 h	140	Sakama & Nishimura (1977)
Rat (male)	unknown	unknown, but uptake by inhalation only	4 h	340	Kimmerle & Lorke (1968)
Rat	80%(?)	vapour whole body	4 h	15	Sasinovich (1968, 1970)
Rat	98%	vapour head only	4 h	> 198	MacDonald (1982)

[a] Solvent C = 0.5% Sorpol 2020 water solution.

5

was not potentiated by pre-treatment (18 h previously) with 30 mg/kg dichlorvos, nor did malathion pre-treatment potentiate the action of dichlorvos.

In vitro studies using human erythrocytes and plasma as ChE sources, with ACh as substrate, indicated no potentiation[a] when dichlorvos was tested in combination with carbaryl, crotoxyphos, phosphamidon, malathion, malaoxon, mevinphos, parathion, paraoxon, physostigmine, and trichlorphon (Carter & Maddux, 1968, 1974).

8.2 Short-term Exposures

8.2.1 Oral

8.2.1.1 Mouse

A 10-week (range-finding) toxicity study was carried out on B6C3F1 mice given 0, 25, 50, 100, 200, or 400 mg dichlorvos/ litre drinking-water. Each group consisted of 12 males and 12 females, except the control group (10 males and 10 females). Growth and mortality were comparable with controls. In a second study, groups of 10 males and 10 females received 400, 1600, 3200, 5000, or 10 000 mg dichlorvos/litre. The animals given the two highest doses died within 2 weeks, while the 1600 and 3200 mg groups showed slight and clear growth depression, respectively, after 10 weeks (Konishi et al., 1981).

8.2.1.2 Rat

For 15 weeks, groups of 15 male and 15 female Charles River rats were fed diets containing 0, 0.1, 1, 10, 100, or 1000 mg dichlorvos (93%)/kg diet, which were freshly prepared once each week. The stability of dichlorvos in the diets was not reported but, in accordance with the 2-year oral rat study (section 8.4.1), it may be assumed that the average concentration of dichlorvos in each diet was approximately 47% of the amount that had been added. There were no deaths or signs of intoxication. Only the rats fed the highest dose exhibited decreased growth rates at the beginning of the study. At termination, no differences were observed in haematology, serum protein, urinalysis, or gross or histopathological examination. In the highest dose group, marked inhibition of ChE activity in plasma, erythrocytes, and brain was noted. In the 100 mg/kg group, only erythrocyte ChE inhibition was observed, and the 10 mg/kg group did not show any ChE inhibition (Witherup et al., 1964).

---

[a] Potentiation is the phenomenon that results in the combined effect of exposure to two or more chemical substances being greater than the sum of the effects that would be produced by each substance separately, as the result of synergistic action.

Daily doses of 3.5 or 7 mg dichlorvos (purity not stated)/kg body weight administered intragastrically to rats for 4 months and 0.7 or 1.4 mg/kg for 12 months caused no deaths. There were signs of intoxication in the 7 mg group, and decreases in food consumption and body weight gain and increases in a number of organ weights were seen in all the groups except the lowest dose group. Inhibition of plasma, erythrocyte, and brain ChE activity was observed in all groups except those given 0.7 mg/kg body weight. The inhibition was time and dose dependent (Sasinovich, 1970).

In a (range-finding) toxicity study, groups of F-344 rats (10 of each sex) were administered 0, 5, 10, 20, 40, or 80 mg/kg body weight, dissolved in 10 ml of drinking-water. During the study six animals died, five of which were in the two highest doses groups (Enomoto, 1981).

Dichlorvos administered orally to rats at a concentration of 70 mg/kg body weight inhibited not only ChE, but also alkaline phosphatase, lactate dehydrogenase, and glutamate dehydrogenase competitively. It increased the activity of glutamic-pyruvic transaminase, but leucine aminopeptidase was not affected (Ellinger, 1985).

Ellinger et al. (1985) also studied the influence of dichlorvos on haematological parameters in acute and short-term toxicity studies. In the acute study 70 mg dichlorvos/kg body weight and in the short-term study 30 mg/kg body weight were administered for 12 weeks. Decreases in haemoglobin, haematocrit, and mean corpuscular haemoglobin concentration were found.

Seven rat mothers were administered different dose levels of dichlorvos (1 g or 10 g/litre distilled water) by stomach tube, and their litters (1 - 12 days old) were nursed for about 21 days, and weaned after 35 days of age. Although doses of 10 and 20 mg/kg body weight did not cause any symptoms of intoxication, the mothers showed significant inhibition of erythrocyte ChE activity. Plasma ChE activity was affected to a lesser extent. Dose levels of 30 and 40 mg/kg body weight caused severe inhibition of erythrocyte ChE, and severe cholinergic symptoms were seen. The symptoms occurred 10 - 20 min after dichlorvos administration and continued for 30 - 90 min, when recovery took place (Tracy et al., 1960).

When pregnant rats were given oral doses of 1 or 5 mg dichlorvos in oil/kg body weight during days 14 - 21 of pregnancy, the plasma ChE activity of the mothers was markedly inhibited, but that of the young (up to 56 days old) resembled the activity in the control. Brain ChE activity did not show any significant inhibition (Zalewska et al., 1977).

8.2.1.3 Rabbit

The progeny of rabbits, treated orally with 6 mg dichlorvos/kg body weight per day for the last 10 days of pregnancy showed a decrease in brain ChE activity and an increase in plasma ChE activity throughout days 1 - 16 of life (Maslinska & Zalewska, 1978).

8.2.1.4 Cat

"Flea collar dermatitis" has been described in cats and dogs wearing dichlorvos-impregnated PVC flea collars. In most cases, flea collar dermatitis is a primary irritant contact dermatitis to dichlorvos. The symptoms may consist of mild local irritation (localized erythema and itching), severe local irritation varying from erythematous alopecia to erosions, ulceration, oedema, and purulent discharges with crusting or, in the most severe cases, generalized dermatitis with secondary pyoderma and systemic illness (Muller, 1970).

Two trials with six and five cats, respectively, were carried out to study the occurrence of contact dermatitis and systemic intoxication. The cats received either a placebo collar or a dichlorvos collar. Two cats received two dichlorvos collars each and each cat was observed for 21 days. In a third trial, four groups of 25 cats were used to study hepatotoxicity. The cats of the different groups were treated as follows. Group 1: placebo collar; Group 2: placebo collar and intraperitoneal treatment with carbon tetrachloride (CCl_4) 7 days later; Group 3: dichlorvos collar; Group 4: dichlorvos collar and intraperitoneal injection of CCl_4 7 days later. Serum glutamic pyruvic transaminase and ChE activity was estimated on day 9 of exposure. In a fourth study, 24 cats were fitted with a placebo collar to test the effect of PVC in relation to the contact dermatitis. PVC did not have an effect. No clear effect of the CCl_4-induced hepatic dystrophy on the detoxification of dichlorvos was found.

The predominant systemic abnormalities recorded in these studies were bone-marrow depression, ataxia, demyelination, and depression. Red cell and plasma ChE activity was severely depressed. Furthermore, contact dermatitis was seen in animals with dichlorvos collars. Ambient temperature and relative humidity may have had a marked influence on these effects, especially in the case of high temperature and low humidity (Bell et al., 1975).

A 90-day study on 90 mongrel cats was carried out to verify the results of Bell et al. (1975) by using a larger number of animals over a longer period. There were three groups of 30 cats; one group with a PVC collar (without dichlorvos), one group with one dichlorvos collar, and the third group with three dichlorvos collars. In this study, in which all relevant parameters were studied, no confirmation of the abnormalities described by Bell et al. (1975) were found, even under conditions of high temperature and low humidity. The only effect was contact dermatitis, but, in this study, this was also found in the PVC collars (Allen et al., 1978).

8.2.1.5 Dog

Groups of three male and three female dogs received equivalents of approximately 0, 0.3, 1, 1.5, or 3 mg dichlorvos (93% in olive oil by gelatin capsule)/kg body weight, daily, for 90 days. No effects were observed on mortality, growth, liver and kidney function, organ weights, haematology, or at gross and histopathological examination. In the two highest dose groups, the dogs showed excitement, increased activity, and aggression. Plasma and erythrocyte ChE activities (measured initially and at intervals of approximately 2 weeks) were normal in the lowest dose group (0.3 mg/kg body weight) but reduced in the other dose groups. Brain ChE activity at termination was reduced only in the highest dose group (Hine, 1962).

8.2.1.6 Pig

Young swine (35 days old) were fed a PVC-resin formulation of dichlorvos (10%) in dosages equivalent to 1, 4, and 16 mg dichlorvos/kg body weight per day in the feed (divided over two daily doses) for 30 days. Body weight gain, blood cell counts, packed-cell volumes, haemoglobin concentrations, plasma glucose, plasma fatty acids, hepatic and muscle glycogen concentrations, plasma and skeletal muscle concentrations of electrolytes, and plasma and pancreatic insulin were all comparable with those of control swine fed a blank PVC formulation. Plasma and erythrocyte ChE activities were significantly inhibited in the 4 and 16 mg/kg groups only (Stanton et al., 1979).

8.2.1.7 Cow

Two cows with suckling calves fed 200 mg dichlorvos/kg grain in their rations showed normal ChE activity in the erythrocytes. However, severe inhibition of ChE activity was found at 500 mg/kg feed (equivalent to 4.5 mg/kg body weight), and a single dose of 27 mg/kg body weight caused cholinergic collapse, followed by rapid recovery. The ChE values in the calves remained normal throughout the 78-day test. Milk from these two cows contained less than 0.08 mg dichlorvos/litre (Tracy et al., 1960).

8.2.2 Dermal

8.2.2.1 Rat

In studies by Dikshith et al. (1976), groups of 48 male rats received daily topical applications of 21.4 mg/kg body weight dichlorvos (96%) in ethanol (control animals received ethanol alone) 5 days per week for 90 days. At intervals of 7, 15, 30, 45, 60, and 90 days, eight test rats and two control rats were sacrificed for histopathological examination of the skin and testes. None of the animals showed signs of intoxication, but ChE activity was not measured. The skin showed no irritation, and no histopathological changes were seen in the testes or skin.

8.2.2.2 Livestock

Spray and dip studies have shown that a concentration of 1% dichlorvos is not toxic for cattle (no further details are available) (Radeleff & Woodard, 1957).

The effect of applying different suspensions (different solvents with and without an emulsifier) of dichlorvos to the skin of cows has been studied. The dose level was 5 mg/kg body weight, increasing after 7 days to 10 mg/kg. Dichlorvos at 5 mg/kg body weight caused a significant decrease in ChE activity in blood serum. The higher dose level additionally produced symptoms of intoxication. No dichlorvos residues were found in milk (Majewski et al., 1978).

Two heifers were washed daily with either a 1% aqueous solution or emulsion of dichlorvos or a 10% suspension of dichlorvos in water (daily application of 1.8 g dichlorvos for 21 days). Two additional heifers were used as controls. The ChE activity levels of the erythrocytes remained at the lower limits of normal variation (Tracy et al., 1960).

8.2.3 Inhalation

8.2.3.1 Experimental animals

In a report by Sasinovich (1968), groups of rats were exposed (whole body) daily for 4 h to average dichlorvos concentrations of 0.11 or 1.1 mg/m^3 for 4 months, to 5.2 mg/m^3 for 2 months, or to 8.2 mg/m^3 for 45 days. The highest dose caused signs of intoxication; two of the eight rats died. Exposure to 5.2 mg/m^3 or more resulted in marked inhibition of ChE activity and disturbance of the blood-sugar curve. In the 0.11 and 1.1 mg/m^3 groups, no significant effects were observed.

Mice, rats, and guinea-pigs, exposed 23 h per day for 28 consecutive days to actual dichlorvos concentrations of 0.03 mg/m^3, did not show gross pathological changes at the end of the study. Inhibition of plasma and brain ChE activity occurred in male mice, male guinea-pigs (plasma only), and female rats (brain only) after a 5-day exposure to 0.14 - 0.15 mg/m^3 dichlorvos (Brown et al., 1968).

Guinea-pigs (P strain) exposed for 7 h per day for 5 consecutive days to an actual concentration of 90 - 120 mg/m^3 dichlorvos suffered no visible effects to their health. Rats (CFE) and mice (CF1) similarly exposed to 50 mg/m^3 were not visibly affected. At concentrations above 50 mg/m^3, the mice became distressed and prolonged exposure to 80 mg/m^3 was frequently lethal. Rats were less severely affected (Stevenson & Blair, 1969).

In studies by Vashkov et al. (1966), 100 mice, 50 rats, 22 rabbits, and 13 cats were exposed to a mixture containing dichlorvos, kerosene, xylene, and freons during a single 2-h exposure or for 2 h per day for 40 days. Three concentrations, 16.5, 45, and 160 mg dichlorvos/m^3, were tested (the median gravimetric diameter of the aerosol particles was about 5 μm). The overall condition of the animals remained normal, and no effects on body weight, clinical chemical blood analyses, blood ChE activity, or respiration rate, or pathological changes were observed. Rabbits developed transient miosis which disappeared at the end of the exposure period.

Mice (20), guinea-pigs (6), sheep (7), calves (39), and a heifer were exposed to an increasing dichlorvos concentration in the air generated by dichlorvos strips (20%). The number of strips was increased each week for 6 weeks, reaching 80 strips per 140 m^3, and was then reduced over the next 6 weeks. During exposure to the recommended number of strips, the dichlorvos concentration in the air was 0.09 - 0.14 mg/m^3. The highest concentration was 2.1 mg/m^3 when the number of strips was 16 times the recommended number. No mortality or signs of intoxication were observed, and mice bore normal litters during the study. The serum ChE activities of the calves and of those handling the animals were within normal values (Henriksson et al., 1971).

When 10 rabbits, 8 cats, and 10 dogs (males and females) were continuously exposed for 8 weeks to dichlorvos concentrations of 0.05 - 0.3 mg/m^3 generated from impregnated PVC-resin strips, no effects were found on general health, behaviour, plasma and erythrocyte ChE activities, or electroencephalographic patterns in the brain of the animals (Walker et al., 1972).

In studies by Coulston & Griffin (1977), four male and four female Rhesus monkeys were continuously exposed to dichlorvos vapour at an average actual concentration of 0.05 mg/m^3 for 3 months. The control group consisted of four males and one female. No adverse effects were observed in appearance, behaviour, or haematological and clinical chemical determinations. Plasma ChE activity was slightly inhibited (up to 28% inhibition), whilst the greatest erythrocyte ChE activity inhibition was 36%. No changes in nerve maximum conduction velocities or muscle-evoked action potentials were induced by the exposure to dichlorvos.

8.2.3.2 Domestic animals

Five horses, exposed continuously to dichlorvos for 22 days in a closed barn that was treated daily with 17 mg dichlorvos/m^3, displayed mild inhibition of erythrocyte ChE activity after 7 days, followed by recovery at 11 - 22 days. However, plasma ChE activity was not changed. The concentration in the barn varied between 0.24 and 1.48 mg/m^3 (Tracy et al., 1960).

The influence on ChE activity in cattle exposed to an impregnated plastic strip containing 20% of dichlorvos has been studied. Red blood cell ChE activity was measured during the 85 days of exposure, and on the 9th day an average inhibition of about 35% was found. After the

37th day the inhibition in ChE activity gradually declined to 20%. No clinical signs were observed (Horvath et al., 1968),

8.2.4 Studies on ChE activity

Groups of 10 young female Sherman rats were fed for 90 days on diets containing 0, 5, 20, 50, 200, 500, or 1000 mg dichlorvos (90%)/kg diet (equivalent to 0, 0.4, 1.5, 3.5, 14.2, 35.7, and 69.9 mg/kg body weight, respectively). Data on the stability of dichlorvos in the diet were not reported. No clinical signs of intoxication were noted. Blood samples were taken from two rats of each group for ChE activity determination on day 3, 11, 60, and 90. In all test groups, a decrease in plasma ChE activity was observed during the first 4 days, gradually returning to normal, except in the rats receiving 14.2 mg/kg body weight or more. At doses above 3.5 mg/kg body weight, erythrocyte ChE activities were decreased throughout the test, but at 3.5 mg/kg body weight, this was only so for the first 30 days of the study. Lower dose levels produced comparable results to those of the control group (Durham et al., 1957).

Thirty-two Rhesus monkeys were treated with 20% pelleted PVC-resin formulations of dichlorvos at dosages ranging from 5 to 80 mg/kg of formulation (equivalent to 1 - 16 mg dichlorvos/kg body weight) daily or 8 and 20 mg/kg of formulation twice daily for 10 - 21 consecutive days. None of the monkeys developed overt signs of intoxication, though they ate less food and had soft faeces. Plasma and erythrocyte ChE activities were reduced by approximately 80% in all animals, and remained inhibited until completion of treatment. Plasma ChE activities returned to normal within approximately 3 weeks, whereas the erythrocyte ChE activities required 50 - 60 days to return to pre-treatment values (Hass et al., 1972).

When groups of five male and five female guinea-pigs (P strain) were given daily applications of 0, 25, 50, or 100 mg dichlorvos (94%)/kg body weight on the shorn skin for 8 days, all the animals survived. A significant dose-dependent inhibition of both plasma and erythrocyte ChE activities occurred in all test groups. Recovery of plasma ChE activities was complete within one week of the last exposure, and that of erythrocyte ChE activities was complete within one week in the females and 2 weeks in the males (Brown & Roberts, 1966).

Three Cynomolgus monkeys were treated daily with dermal doses of 50, 75, and 100 mg/kg body weight technical dichlorvos in xylene for 5 days per week until the animals died (after 8, 10, and 4 doses, respectively). Symptoms of intoxication appeared in all monkeys, beginning 10 - 20 min after administration of the first dose. The erythrocyte ChE activity decreased rapidly and remained severely inhibited for the period of the study, while plasma ChE activities fluctuated throughout the study (Durham et al., 1957).

When male and female mice, rats, and guinea-pigs were exposed continuously by inhalation for 5 consecutive days to actual concentrations of 0, 0.14 - 0.15, or 1.1 - 1.3 mg/m^3 dichlorvos, no overt signs of intoxication were observed. In the high exposure groups, plasma, erythrocyte, and brain ChE activities were inhibited in all three species. Plasma ChE was the most sensitive in all three species, with up to 70% inhibition in the female mice. The greatest inhibition of brain ChE activity (30%) was found in mice (Brown et al., 1968).

The effects of dichlorvos vapour inhalation on AChE activity was investigated in the rat. Exposure to dichlorvos concentrations of 0.8 and 1.8 mg/m^3 for 3 days reduced AChE activity in the bronchial tissue (50 - 60% of control) but did not produce any changes in blood AChE activity. However, at 4.3 mg/m^3, blood AChE activity also declined (38% of control). In histochemical preparations, staining of the bronchial glands and smooth muscles revealed reduced enzyme activity even at the lowest dose (0.2 mg/m^3) tested. At this concentration, no inhibition of bronchial homogenate ChE was observed (Schmidt et al., 1975, 1979). The significance of bronchial ChE inhibition is not clear.

Male mice were continuously exposed to actual concentrations of 0 or 0.03 mg dichlorvos/m^3 for 28 consecutive days. Weekly assays of ChE activities showed that brain ChE activity was slightly inhibited (less than 20%) on the 28th day only, but plasma and erythrocyte ChE activities were not significantly inhibited (Brown et al., 1968).

Rabbits exposed to an average concentration of 1 mg dichlorvos/m^3 (0.8 - 1.3 mg/m^3) for 4 h per day for 4 months showed up to 30% inhibition of serum and erythrocyte ChE activities during the study. However, cats similarly exposed did not show significant inhibition (Sasinovich, 1968).

Rats and monkeys were exposed for 2 weeks in an inhalation chamber sprayed once with an emulsion of dichlorvos. The initial air concentration was 6 mg dichlorvos/m^3, decreasing over a few days to about 0.1 - 0.2 mg/m^3. No signs of intoxication were seen. The plasma and erythrocyte ChE activities of the monkeys decreased to approximately 50% of pre-exposure levels, but rapid recovery took place after cessation of exposure. Comparable results were obtained when rats and monkeys were continuously exposed for up to 7 days to a maximum air concentration of 2.2 mg/m^3. However, continuous exposure for 4 days to 0.27 mg/m^3 did not produce any effect on ChE activity (Durham et al., 1957).

Groups of two monkeys were exposed to dichlorvos vapour 2 h per day for 4 consecutive days. With concentrations up to 0.7 mg/m^3, no change in plasma or erythrocyte ChE activity was noted, while 1.2 - 3.3 mg/m^3 caused a slight decrease in plasma ChE activity, and 7.5 - 18 mg/m^3 (mean: 13 mg/m^3) resulted in miosis and a pronounced inhibition (40 - 70%) of plasma and erythrocyte ChE activities (Witter et al., 1961).

Groups of 10 chickens were exposed to dichlorvos vapour from a varying number of strips (20% dichlorvos) continually or intermittently for 3 weeks. Exposure to a single strip in a room of 33 m^3 (either interrupted or for 16 h every day) produced no significant effect on plasma or brain ChE activity. Exposure to more than one strip (2 - 5) resulted in up to 50% inhibition of plasma ChE activity and approximately 40% inhibition of brain ChE activity. Dichlorvos aerosol sprays (0.7% dichlorvos) showed that daily excessive spraying for 6 seconds, 8 times per day, for 5 days, did not produce significant ChE inhibition. However, a significant decrease in plasma ChE activity was found when the study lasted for 21 days (Rauws & van Logten, 1973).

Three studies were carried out to determine the effect on the laying performance of hens given dichlorvos in the feed for 4 weeks. Plasma AChE levels were reduced by 70% at 20, 30, or 40 mg dichlorvos/kg diet, although there was no clear influence on food consumption, egg production, egg weight, or hatchability at these doses. At 80 mg/kg diet, a decrease in food consumption and in egg production was seen, the latter being a consequence, possibly, of the former (Pym et al., 1984).

8.3 Skin and Eye Irritation; Sensitization

In the skin sensitization assay procedure of Stevens (flank/flank technique), 1% dichlorvos in olive oil produced no visible effects in male albino guinea-pigs. Negative results were also obtained when five components of formulated dichlorvos/ PVC products were assayed for their skin sensitization potential (Kodama, 1968).

A primary skin irritation test on dichlorvos was performed by using male New Zealand white rabbits. Irritation observed on the skin after the application of 5 - 20% water solutions of dichlorvos was relatively severe compared with that caused by other organophosphorus insecticides (Arimatsu et al., 1977).

In order to study the allergenicity of dichlorvos, the guinea-pig maximization test was used. Threshold limit values of primary irritancy tested on the skin of guinea-pigs (Hartley strain) were 2% or more. In the maximization test, 0.05 and 0.5% were used. With 0.5%, 35% of the animals showed slight or discrete erythema. The allergenicity rating as determined by the Kligman test was moderate. In combination with methidathion, dichlorvos showed a stronger reaction, indicating cross-sensitization (Fujita, 1985).

8.4 Long-term Exposure

8.4.1 Oral

8.4.1.1 Rat

In studies by Witherup et al. (1967, 1971), groups of 40 male and 40 female weanling CD rats were fed diets containing nominal concentrations of 0, 0.1, 1, 10, 100, or 500 mg dichlorvos (93%)/kg diet for 2 years. Five males and five females from each group were sacrificed after 6, 12, and 18 months, and analysis of diet samples showed a considerable loss of dichlorvos. This was associated with a gradual increase in DCA concentration which ranged in the different groups from 0.014 to 28.6 mg/kg diet. The average actual concentrations of dichlorvos in each diet were 0, 0.047, 0.467, 4.67, 46.7, and 234 mg/kg diet (equivalent to approximately 0, 0.0025, 0.025, 0.25, 2.5, and 12.5 mg/kg body weight). There were no signs of intoxication, and no effects were seen on behaviour, mortality rate, food consumption, weight gain, organ weights, haematology, or urinalysis. Plasma and erythrocyte ChE activities were decreased throughout the study in the two highest dose groups compared with controls, but brain ChE activity was decreased in the highest dose group only. Histological examination of major organs revealed hepatocellular fatty vacuolization in the group with 234 mg/kg and in some of the animals with 46.7 mg/kg diet. No effect was seen on serum total proteins or albumin:globulin ratio, or on hexobarbital sleeping time. It can be concluded that the actual average concentration of 4.7 mg/kg diet (equivalent to approximately 0.25 mg/kg body weight) was without significant effect on any of the measured parameters. The tumour incidence was comparable with that of the control group.

8.4.1.2 Dog

Groups of three male and three female beagle dogs were fed diets containing 0, 0.1, 1, 10, 100, or 500 mg dichlorvos (93%)/kg diet for 2 years, the average actual concentrations being 0, 0.09, 0.32, 3.2, 32, and 256 mg dichlorvos/kg diet (equivalent to 0, 0.002, 0.008, 0.08, 0.8, and 6.4 mg/kg body weight). The average DCA concentration in the diets with 10, 100, and 500 mg dichlorvos/kg diet was 0.6, 6.4, and 20 mg/kg diet. No effects were seen on general appearance, survival, food consumption, weight gain, haematology, or urinalysis. However, erythrocyte ChE was inhibited at dose levels of 3.2 mg/kg diet or more, and plasma ChE activity was inhibited at the two highest dose levels. Recovery to control values took place at the end of the feeding period. Brain ChE activity, measured at the end of the study, was similar to that of the controls, and liver weights were increased in both sexes in the 256 mg/kg diet group. Histological examination of major organs revealed slight dose-related alterations in the hepatic cells of one female in the 3.2 mg/kg diet group, and greater alterations at higher doses. No differences were seen in serum alkaline phosphatase, transaminase activities, total serum proteins, or albumin:globulin ratios. The actual average concentration of 0.32 mg/kg diet (equivalent to 0.008 mg/kg body weight) was without effect (Jolley et al., 1967; Witherup et al., 1971).

8.4.2 Inhalation

8.4.2.1 Rat

When groups of 50 male and 50 female weanling CFE rats were exposed for 23 h per day to air concentrations of 0, 0.05, 0.5, or 5 mg dichlorvos (97%)/m^3 air (actual concentrations: 0, 0.05, 0.48, and 4.7 mg/m^3) for 2 years, body weight gain was reduced in the two highest dose groups. After 2 years of exposure, plasma and erythrocyte ChE activities were significantly reduced in the two highest dose groups, but in the case of brain ChE activity, only in the highest group. No effects attributable to dichlorvos were seen on appearance, food consumption, haematological or blood chemistry values, or organ weights, or upon gross or microscopic examination. Ultrastructural examinations of bronchi and alveoli of rats exposed to 0 or 5 mg/m^3 showed no differences between the two groups.

In connection with a reported correlation between brain ACh concentration and the inhibition of brain ChE activity following acute exposure to organophosphorus compounds, the brain tissue of three female rats per group was examined for ACh and choline concentrations. The dose level of 0.05 mg dichlorvos/m^3 was without effect on any of the measured parameters (Blair et al., 1976). It should be noted that in this study the rats were not only exposed by inhalation but also via their food, drinking-water, and by grooming. This resulted in additional oral ingestion of dichlorvos (Stevenson & Blair, 1977).

8.5 Reproduction, Embryotoxicity, and Teratogenicity

8.5.1 Reproduction

In a 3-generation reproduction study, weanling CD rats (six groups of 30 animals) were fed dichlorvos (93%) at nominal concentrations of 0, 0.1, 1, 10, 100, or 500 mg/kg diet, prepared freshly each week. The stability of dichlorvos in the diets was not reported but, in accordance with the 2-year oral rat study (section 8.4.1.1), it was assumed that the average concentration of dichlorvos was approximately 47% of the nominal concentrations (equivalent to 0, 0.0025, 0.025, 0.25, 2.5, and 12.5 mg/kg body weight). No effects on fertility, number and size of litters, body weight, or viability of the pups were found. Gross and histopathological examination of 7-day-old pups from F_{1a} and F_{2a} litters did not reveal any abnormalities (Witherup et al., 1965, 1971).

Oral treatment of rats with 5.6 mg/kg body weight and rabbits with 6 mg/kg body weight during the last trimester of pregnancy had no effect on offspring weight and development. However, the cerebral cortices from the 1-day-old rabbits were less mature than those of control rabbits, probably due to maternal toxicity (Dambska et al., 1978, 1979).

Dambska & Maslinska (1982) observed impairment of the development of the brain of rabbits dosed orally with 9 mg/kg body weight per day from days 5 to 16 of life, the period of myelination.

8.5.1.1 Effects on testes

In studies by Krause & Homolo (1972, 1974), three groups of 14 male NMRI/Han mice received either a single oral dose of 40 mg dichlorvos/kg body weight, daily oral doses of 10 mg dichlorvos (in olive oil)/kg for 18 consecutive days, or daily oral doses of 0.5 ml olive oil for 18 days, respectively. On days 9, 18, 27, 36, 54, and 63, two animals from each group were killed and their testes examined histologically. Severe disturbances of spermatogenesis were observed in both test groups; damaged seminiferous tubules were also seen and the supporting Sertoli cells were damaged. In addition, there was an increase in the number and hypertrophy of the Leydig cells. No explanation could be offered for these effects.

A similar study was carried out on three groups of 16 male juvenile Wistar rats. The rats received either 20 mg dichlorvos (in olive oil)/kg body weight on days 4 and 5, 10 mg dichlorvos (in olive oil)/kg daily from days 4 to 23, or 0.1 ml olive oil daily from days 4 to 23 of life. On days 6, 12, 18, 26, 34, and 50 of life, two rats from each group were sacrificed. Histological examination of the testes showed slight reduction in the number of the spermatogenic cells and Leydig cells. It was assumed that a reduction in testosterone synthesis resulted in damage to the spermatogenic cells. All the changes were reversed by the 50th day (Krause et al., 1976; Xing-Shu, 1983).

In order to examine the cause of the observed effect on the spermatogenic and Leydig cells, the study was repeated with, in addition, measurement of testosterone levels in serum and testes. The testosterone concentrations in the testes, and leutinizing hormone (LH) and follicle stimulating hormone (FSH) levels in serum were similar in the presence or absence of dichlorvos (Krause, 1977). However, the use of adult rats and a different dosing regimen prevented a strict comparison with the earlier study by Krause et al. (1976).

In studies by Fujita et al. (1977), 55 male Wistar rats (aged 5 months) were orally administered dichlorvos at levels of 5 or 10 mg/kg body weight every other day for 8 weeks. The rats were divided into five groups, and one group of rats was killed every 4 weeks to study the changes in several organs, including the testes. About 200 individual seminiferous tubules were examined in each rat. No change was seen in body weight gain or testes weight. The score values of the seminal cellular system decreased after 4 - 8 weeks of treatment, but were restored 8 weeks after the end of treatment.

8.5.1.2 Effect on estrous cycle

Timmons et al. (1975) reported studies on female rats which were exposed to an atmosphere containing 2.4 mg dichlorvos/m^3 generated from a dichlorvos strip placed on top of each cage. Exposure was continuous from the birth of the first litter until the estrous cycle began again. Controls were housed in a separate room. A significant mean delay of 10 days in the onset of the estrous cycle, compared with that of controls, was observed. However, the significance of the results was complicated by different housing conditions.

8.5.1.3 Domestic animals

In studies by Bazer et al. (1969), sows were fed dichlorvos (9% in resin pellets) at the level of 800 mg per animal per day beginning 21 days before breeding and continuing through gestation. No significant differences in the numbers born alive or dead, the litter weight, number weaned, or individual weaning weights were observed.

In a further study, dichlorvos was added to the rations of pregnant sows at the level of 0 or 800 mg per animal per day. Resin pellets containing 9% dichlorvos were fed either from 3 weeks before breeding and throughout gestation, or from 18 to 56 days before parturition. Data were collected from a total of 681 dams, representing eight replicates over a period of 2 years. The dichlorvos-treated groups scored consistently higher for individual farrowing weights, litter farrowing weights, number weaned, individual weaning weights, and litter weaning weights, and less consistently, for the percentage of live births (Batte et al., 1969).

When dichlorvos (as a PVC-resin formulation) was administered to sows in doses ranging from 4 to 13 mg/kg body weight per day for the last 21 - 30 days of gestation, the average farrowing interval for the live-born piglets was shorter in treated than in control animals. There was also a dose-related increase in the mean birth weight of live-born piglets from the dichlorvos-treated sows, while the incidence of still births was lower than in controls (Bunding et al., 1972).

In studies by Collins et al. (1971), male and female swine were fed for up to 3 years on diets containing a PVC-resin formulation at 0, 200, 250, 288, 400, or 500 mg dichlorvos/kg diet, and for at least 6 months prior to initial breeding. Two generations were raised, and no effects were observed on number or size of litters, survival or growth rate of offspring, urinalysis, haematology, hepatic and renal function, physical structure, or calcium and phosphorus content of the femoral bone, or in appearance during gross and microscopic examination. Organ weights were normal except in the case of the liver, which was generally increased. Whole blood ChE activity was inhibited and brain ChE activity was slightly reduced, but no clinical evidence of neurophysiological impairment was observed.

In studies reported by Stanton et al. (1979), pregnant sows were given PVC-resin formulations of dichlorvos (10%) in the diet at a daily dose of 0, 5, or 25 mg dichlorvos/kg body weight (divided between two doses per day) during the last one-third of pregnancy (or 30 days). Only about 50% of the total dichlorvos was released from this resin in the gastrointestinal tract. All pigs were born alive, and their birth weight was similar to that of control animals. In the group given 25 mg/kg body weight, plasma and erythrocyte ChE activities were markedly inhibited (80 and 90%, respectively) in the sows, but not in the newborn pigs. No changes in the packed cell volume or haemoglobin concentration of the sows or their piglets were observed.

In a limited test reported by Darrow (1973), dichlorvos-impregnated collars did not have any adverse effects on pregnant female goats or later on their newborn young. Also, blood ChE activity was not inhibited in either the nannies or the kids over a period of several weeks. The acceptance of treated kids by the mothers was normal.

A pregnant non-lactating Holstein-Friesian cow was fed a nominal concentration of 6.2 mg dichlorvos/kg body weight per day in the daily ration from days 152 to 286 of pregnancy. A normal calf was delivered (Macklin & Ribelin, 1971).

A herd of 54 dairy cows (two-thirds carrying calves) was accidently sprayed with dichlorvos, resulting in a dosage of 50 mg dichlorvos/kg body weight. All the animals showed symptoms of intoxication and some had convulsions. However, they all recovered within a few hours, with no abortions or other adverse effects except a temporary diminution in milk production (Knapp & Graden, 1964).

When three pregnant sows were fed 8.5 mg dichlorvos/kg body weight per day (as PVC-resin formulation) from days 41 to 70 of pregnancy, the blood ChE activity of the sows was markedly inhibited, but no demonstrable teratogenic effects or functional abnormalities in the piglets were found (Wrathall et al., 1980).

8.5.2 Embryotoxicity and teratogenicity

8.5.2.1 Oral

In studies by Schwetz et al. (1979), CF1 mice and New Zealand rabbits were given maximum tolerated doses of dichlorvos (96%) in corn oil by gavage, at levels of 60 and 5 mg/kg body weight, respectively, from days 6 to 15 and days 6 to 18 of gestation, respectively. Except for an increased number of resorptions in rabbits, no significant effect was observed on the mean number of live fetuses per litter, or on fetal body measurements. There were no gross visceral or skeletal alterations. In mice, no abnormalities were found.

Carson (1969) reported studies on a total of 168 New Zealand rabbits, divided into 10 groups containing 15 - 26 animals. One group received lactose capsules, three groups different PVC-placebo capsules, and three groups PVC capsules containing 18, 54, or 93 mg dichlorvos/animal. These capsules were provided twice daily, so that the equivalent daily intake was 12, 36, or 62 mg/kg body weight, respectively. The rabbits received 12 or 36 mg dichlorvos/kg body weight on days 6 - 18 of gestation, or 62 mg/kg body weight on days 6 - 11 of gestation. Fetuses were obtained by Caesarian section. Maternal mortality was increased in the highest dichlorvos group, and the incidences of *in utero* and neonatal toxicity were also increased (but not significantly) in the 62 mg group, compared with those in the control groups. The fetal mortality was not clearly indicative of any marked toxic effects other than those involving the dam, since whole litters were not involved. Extensive skeletal and soft tissue examinations were carried out on all viable neonates, but no adverse effects on bone formation, articulation, or degree of ossification were found in the dichlorvos groups. No teratogenic effects were observed.

When pregnant rabbits were given oral doses of PVC-resin formulations during the critical days of organogenesis, doses of 34 mg dichlorvos/kg body weight or more were found to cause maternal toxicity. With doses of 12 mg/kg body weight or less, no significant effect on nidation, *in utero* survival, or neonatal survival was found. No evidence of teratogenic changes was observed on gross, visceral, or skeletal examination of the fetuses (Vogin et al., 1971).

The effect of dichlorvos on embryonal and fetal development in thyroparathyroidectomized, thyroxine-treated, and euthyroid control rats has been investigated. On days 8 - 15 of gestation, 25 mg dichlorvos/kg body weight per day was administered orally to pregnant Charles River rats, and a slight decrease in fetal weight in all groups was observed. No gross, visceral, or skeletal anomalies of the fetuses were found as a result of dichlorvos administration to rats with altered thryoid status (Baksi, 1978).

8.5.2.2 Inhalation

In studies by Thorpe et al. (1972), rats of E strain and Dutch rabbits were exposed (23 h per day, 7 days per week) throughout pregnancy to nominal concentrations of 0, 0.25, 1.25, or 6.25 mg dichlorvos/m^3. In an additional study, groups of 20 pregnant rabbits were exposed to nominal concentrations of 2 or 4 mg dichlorvos/m^3. Maternal deaths occurred in the rabbits exposed to 2 mg/m^3 or more, and ChE activities in plasma, erythrocytes, and brain were markedly inhibited in both species exposed to 1.25 mg/m^3 or more. There was no indication of any dichlorvos-related teratogenic effects.

When CF1 mice and New Zealand rabbits were exposed to dichlorvos at an average actual concentration of 4 mg/m^3 for 7 h per day from days 6 to 15 and from days 6 to 18 of gestation, respectively, no significant effect on the mean number of live fetuses per litter, the incidence or distribution of resorptions, or on fetal body measurements was noted. No gross, visceral, or skeletal alterations were observed (Schwetz et al., 1979).

8.5.2.3 Intraperitoneal

Kimbrough & Gaines (1968) reported a study on female Sherman rats given a single intraperitoneal injection of 0 or 15 mg dichlorvos (in peanut oil)/kg body weight on day 11 of pregnancy. The treated dams showed toxic signs and weight loss. On day 20, the fetuses were removed. There was no adverse effect on litter size, resorptions, number of dead fetuses per litter, or average weight of fetuses, but 3 out of 41 fetuses had omphaloceles. This latter finding, observed at a maternally toxic dose, is not in agreement with the other teratology studies or the 3-generation reproduction study.

8.5.3 Résumé of reproduction, embryotoxicity, and teratogenicity studies

A 3-generation study on rats, fed dichlorvos at dose levels of up to 500 mg/kg diet, did not show any effects on fertility, number and size of litters, body weight, or viability of the pups.

In studies on mice and rats, high dose levels of dichlorvos (a single dose of 40 mg/kg body weight or multiple doses of 5 or 10 mg/kg body weight) induced disturbances in spermatogenesis, characterized by damage to the seminiferous tubules and Sertoli cells and by hypertrophy and increase in the number of Leydig cells. It was assumed, but not confirmed, that testosterone synthesis was partially inhibited. After dichlorvos treatment ceased, recovery was complete within about 2 months.

A number of reproduction studies on domestic animals, mainly sows, have been carried out. Levels of 500 mg/kg diet for 3 years had no effect on fertility. Inhibition of ChE activity in the sows, but not in the newborn pigs, was induced by 25 mg/kg body weight. No teratogenic effects were seen.

Teratogenicity studies on rats and rabbits, orally administered 62 mg/kg body weight during gestation, revealed symptoms of intoxication and significant inhibition of ChE in the parent rabbits. Except for an increased number of resorptions, no significant effect on the mean number of live fetuses per litter or evidence of a teratogenic effect was noted during gross, visceral, or skeletal examination.

There were no teratogenic effects after rats inhaled 6.25 mg dichlorvos/m^3 during gestation, though maternal deaths occurred. Mice and rabbits exposed to 4 mg/m^3 on days 6 - 18 of gestation did not show any effects.

8.6 Mutagenicity and Related End-Points

8.6.1 Methylating reactivity

In a quantitative colour test for alkylating agents, dichlorvos gave a positive response, whereas the metabolites desmethyldichlorvos, dimethylphosphate, dichloroethanol, DCA, and dichloroacetic acid all gave negative results (Bedford & Robinson, 1972).

8.6.1.1 In vitro studies

Lawley et al. (1974) have shown that methylation by dichlorvos of DNA and RNA, using either isolated nucleic acids, *Escherichia coli* cells, or human tumour HeLa cells, broadly resembled that by methylmethanesulfonate (MMS) rather than methylation by *N*-methyl-*N*-nitrosourea. In *E. coli* cells, 3-methyladenine, the principal minor product in methylated DNA apart from 7-methylguanine, was not detected, whereas it was present when pre-isolated DNA was methylated. The overall extent of methylation achieved in cells was small. Specific excision of 3-methyladenine was indicated in *E. coli* cells (Lawley et al., 1974).

Labelled 7-methylguanine was present in both DNA and RNA isolated from *E. coli* exposed to ^{3}H-dichlorvos. The methylating capability of dichlorvos was less, by a factor of 10 - 100, than that of strongly genotoxic methylating compounds (Wennerberg & Löfroth, 1974). Alkylation by dichlorvos of calf thymus DNA, resulting in the formation of *N*-7-methylguanine, was reported by Löfroth (1970).

Shooter (1975) has applied the test for chain breaks in RNA to the interaction of dichlorvos with bacteriophage R_{17}. Breaks in the RNA chain result from the hydrolysis of phosphotriesters and are thus a measure of the extent of O-alkylation and of the S_N1-type mechanism of the reaction. The results so far suggest that the existence of O-alkylation, as shown by degradation following phosphotriester formation, does correlate with mutagenicity. Incubation of bacteriophage R_{17} with 0 - 100 mmol dichlorvos/litre for 90 h did not result in methylation of the phosphate group of the RNA to any significant extent.

8.6.1.2 In vivo studies

Reviews of the literature on alkylating agents including dichlorvos have been made by Bedford & Robinson (1972), Lohs et al. (1976), and Hemminki (1983).

In studies in which mice were given intraperitoneal injections of methyl-^{14}C-dichlorvos (1.9 µmol/kg body weight), the degree of alkylation of guanine-*N*-7 in DNA isolated from soft tissues amounted to 8 x 10^{-13} mol methyl/g DNA. From this, a rate of clearance of approximately 1.4 min was estimated (Segerbäck, 1981; Segerbäck & Ehrenberg, 1981). DNA and RNA from the total soft tissues of male CFE rats exposed to atmospheres containing 0.064 mg methyl-^{14}C-dichlorvos/m^3 for 12 h did not show methylation of the N-7 atom of guanine moieties. The exposure period constituted a significant fraction of the half-life of the 7-methylguanine moieties in DNA. It was concluded that dichlorvos does not pose a methylating hazard to mammalian DNA *in vivo* (Wooder et al., 1977; Wooder & Wright, 1981).

The excretion of labelled 7-methyl guanine in the urine by NMRI mice and R rats injected intraperitoneally with methyl-^{14}C-dichlorvos, or exposed by inhalation for 2 h (mice only), was reported by Löfroth & Wennerberg (1974) and Wennerberg & Löfroth (1974). In rat urine, labelled 3-methyladenine and 1-methylnicotinamide were also detected (Löfroth & Wennerberg, 1974). According to the authors, these results demonstrate the dichlorvos-induced methylation of guanine and adenine moieties in nucleic acids.

However, the administration of radiolabelled adenine and guanine to otherwise untreated rats gave rise to the excretion of radiolabelled methylated purines in the urine. Therefore, the detection of radiolabelled purines, *per se*, in the urine of animals exposed to methyl-labelled methylating agents, does not constitute evidence for the methylation of the purine moieties of nucleosides or nucleic acids by methylating agents (Wooder et al., 1978). Moreover, the results of metabolic studies have demonstrated the existence of a natural biosynthetic pathway whereby the methyl carbon atoms of dichlorvos can, with partial retention of hydrogen, become incorporated into the heterocyclic rings and the methyl groups of urinary 7-methylguanine after entering 1-C pools, *in vivo*. The results of preliminary studies suggest the existence of a similar pathway for the production of urinary 3-methyladenine (Wright et al., 1979).

Wooder & Creedy (1979) described a study on rats which investigated the DNA-damaging potential of dichlorvos when administered as a single intraperitoneal dose. Alkaline sucrose gradient profiles of rat liver DNA showed that whereas MMS (a positive control) shifted the DNA profile, dichlorvos at 10 mg/kg body weight (the maximum dose consistent with survival) had no effect.

8.6.1.3 Discussion of methylating reactivity

Many alkylation tests and *in vivo* and *in vitro* mutagenicity studies have been carried out with dichlorvos. It has been demonstrated that dichlorvos has alkylating properties, and has been suggested from some studies that the *in vivo* alkylating potential of dichlorvos is similar to that of some known mutagens. However, this concern is misplaced since alternative reactions were not considered (WHO, 1986b). The phosphorus atom is markedly more electron-deficient and susceptible to attack by nucleophiles than the alkyl carbon atom. Analysis by Bedford & Robinson (1972) of the data of Löfroth et al. (1969) revealed that the proposed rates of alkylation by potent nucleophiles were probably combined rates of phosphorylation and alkylation, and that phosphorylation was the totally dominant reaction in the case of the hydroxide ion. The comparison with known mutagens is therefore inappropriate. Two factors detract further from the toxicological significance of the alkylation studies. The first is that mammalian tissues (plasma, liver, etc.) contain active A-esterase enzymes, which catalyse the phosphorylation of water by the organophosphorus esters. Viewed inversely, these A-esterases catalyse the hydrolysis of the organophosphorus esters, thereby rapidly reducing circulating levels of hazardous material. Secondly, the comparative rate of reaction of most of these esters with AChE is many orders of magnitude greater than the rate of alkylation by the typical nucleophile 4-nitrobenzyl-pyridine: for dichlorvos, the ratio of rates was 1×10^7 in favour of the inhibitory phosphorylation of AChE (Aldridge & Johnson, 1977). It follows that, at low exposure levels, *in vivo* phosphorylation of AChE and other esterases will be the dominant reaction, with negligible uncatalysed alkylation of nucleic acid. Indeed, no such alkylation has been detected in sensitive *in vivo* studies designed to check this point (Wooder et al., 1977).

8.6.2 Mutagenicity

Reviews of the existing literature have been published by Wild (1975), Fishbein (1976, 1981, 1982), Leonard (1976), IARC (1979), Sternberg (1979), Ramel et al. (1980), Lafontaine et al. (1981), Ramel (1981), and Wildemauwe et al. (1983).

8.6.2.1 In vitro studies

(a) *Microorganisms*

Numerous mutagenicity studies using bacteria and fungi as test organisms have been carried out (Table 17). In most of the studies, only one dichlorvos concentration, often a high one, was tested, sometimes resulting in low survival of the test organism. A dose-response relationship was established in the few tests where a range of concentrations was used. The results indicate that dichlorvos induces base substitutions in bacteria and mitotic gene conversion in yeast. The alkylating properties of dichlorvos (section 8.6.1) are most probably the cause of the mutagenic action. This was the conclusion of Bridges et al. (1973) from tests using both MMS and dichlorvos with *E. coli* strains deficient at four different repair loci.

In *Aspergillus nidulans*, dichlorvos has been found to induce point mutations to 8-azaguanine resistance and a high frequency of mitotic crossing-over and non-disjunction (Aulicino et al., 1976; Bignami et al., 1976, 1977; Morpurgo et al., 1979). No mutagenic activity using *A. nidulans* was found after incubating *Nicotiana alata* cell cultures with dichlorvos for 21 days (simulating *in vitro* plant metabolism). This confirms the rapid metabolism of dichlorvos (Benigni et al., 1979).

The mutagenicity of dichlorvos has been extensively studied in Japan, (Kawachi et al., 1980). Dichlorvos induced gene mutation in *Salmonella typhimurium* TA100 as well as *E. coli* strains in the absence of rat-liver S9 mix.

Dichlorvos (0.5 - 2 mg/ml) causes random strand breakage, repairable by DNA polymerase I, in *E. coli* pol A as detected by the alkaline sucrose sedimentation method. When pol$^+$ bacteria and high concentrations of dichlorvos (0.2 - 0.4%) were used, an all-or-none breakdown of DNA molecules to fragments of very low relative molecular mass occurred which correlated well with lethality. It has been suggested that the major DNA damage resulting from dichlorvos treatment arises indirectly through alkylation of other cellular constituents, this leading to uncontrolled nuclease attack on DNA. However, discontinuities in newly-synthesized DNA and mutagenesis following

Table 17. Mutagenicity tests on microorganisms

Organism/strain	Dose	Type of test	Metabolic activation	Result	Reference
Bacillus subtilis					
H17 rec^+	0.02 ml of	plate	none	-	Shirasu et al. (1976)
M45 rec^-	10% solution	plate	none	+	
Citrobacter freundii					
425	0.1%	fluctuation	none	weak +	Voogd et al. (1972)
	0.05%		none	-	
Enterobacter aerogenes					
6	0.1%	fluctuation	none	weak +	Voogd et al. (1972)
Escherichia coli					
B	5 - 25 mmol/litre 1- to 10-h exposure	liquid induction streptomycin-resistant mutants	none	weak + (dose- and exposure-time related)	Wild (1973)
B/r WP2	22.6 mmol/litre	plate reversion	none	+	Moriya et al. (1978)
			S9 mix	+	
			L-cysteine	+	
CM 561, 571, 611	5 µl	plate reversion	none	-	Hanna & Dyer (1975)
K12HfrH	0.1%	fluctuation	none	weak +	Voogd et al. (1972)
K12(5-MT)	3.3×10^{-4} mol/litre	plate	none	+	Mohn (1973)

Table 17 (contd).

Organism/strain	Dose	Type of test	Metabolic activation	Result	Reference
Escherichia coli (contd).					
WP2	micro drop analytical and technical grade, aqueous solution	plate	none	-	Dean (1972a)
WP2 try$^-$	approximately 20 mm^2 dichlorvos strip	plate	none	+	Ashwood-Smith et al. (1972)
WP2 try$^-$ hcr$^-$ and hcr$^+$	20 - 25 μl of 50% emulsifiable concentrate	spot back mutation	none	+	Nagy et al. (1975)
	0.1 ml of a 5% solution	plate reversion	none	+	Shirasu et al. (1976)
WP2 hcr	unknown (up to 5000 μg/plate)	plate reversion	none	+	Moriya et al. (1983)
WP2 uvrA, WP 67	ca 5 μl	plate reversion	none	+	Hanna & Dyer (1975)
Klebsiella pneumoniae	0.1%; 0.05%	fluctuation	none	weak +	Voogd et al. (1972)
Neurospora crassa ad-3	exposed to air containing dichlorvos (strip)	plate	none	-	Michalek & Brockman (1969)
Pseudomonas aeruginosa PAO 38	0.08 mol/litre	liquid reversion	none	+	Dyer & Hanna (1973)

Table 17 (contd)

Saccharomyces cerevisiae					
D4 (ade2 and trp5)	4 mg/ml 2 mg/ml	plate mitotic gene conversion	none	+ -	Dean et al. (1972)
D4 (ade2 and trp5)	19 mmol	liquid mitotic gene conversion	none	+	Fahrig (1973, 1974)
Salmonella typhimurium					
64-320	0.05%; 0.1%	suspension	none	+	Voogd et al. (1972)
TA 98	20 or 40 mmol	plate	S9 male mice	-	Braun et al. (1982)
	up to 5000 μg	plate reversion	none	-	Moriya et al. (1983)
TA 100	20 or 40 mmol	plate	S9 male mice	(+) low survival	Braun et al. (1982)
	up to 5000 μg	plate reversion	none	+	Moriya et al. (1983)
TA 1530	5 μl	plate	none	+	Hanna & Dyer (1975)
TA 1535	5 μl	plate	none	+	Hanna & Dyer (1975)
	0.1 ml of a 5% solution	plate	none	+	Shirasu et al. (1976)
	0.1 ml of a 5% solution	plate	none S9 mix L-cysteine	+ - -	Moriya et al. (1978)
	2800 μg	plate (spot)	S9 male rat	-	Carere et al. (1976, 1978a,b)
	1.5 mg/ml	liquid	none	+	Carere et al. (1978a,b)

Table 17 (contd)

Organism/strain	Dose	Type of test	Metabolic activation	Result	Reference
Salmonella typhimurium (contd).					
TA 1535	20 or 40 mmol	plate	S9 male mice	-	Braun et al. (1982)
TA 1536, 1537, 1538	0.1 ml of a 5% solution	plate	none	-	Shirasu et al. (1976)
TA 1536, 1537, 1538	2800 µg	plate (spot)	S9 male rat	-	Carere et al. (1976, 1978a,b)
	20 or 40 µg	plate	S9 male mice	-	Braun et al. (1982)
	up to 5000 µg	plate	none	-	Moriya et al. (1983)
his C117	0.03 mol	liquid	none	+	Dyer & Hanna (1973)
LT2 his C117, his G 46	5 µl	plate	none	-	Hanna & Dyer (1975)
Schizosaccharomyces pombe					
ade6	1.5 - 14 mmol	plate	+	+	Gilot-Delhalle et al. (1983)
Serratia marcescens					
Hy alpha 13, alpha 21	25 mg/ml	plate (spot)	none	alpha 13 + alpha 21 -	Dean (1972a)
	50, 100 mg/ml	plate (spot)	none	+	Dean (1972a)
	saturated aqueous solution	plate (spot)	none	+	Dean (1972a)
Streptomyces coelicolor					
A 3(2) his A1	5600 µg	spot	none	+	Carere et al. (1976, 1978a,b)

dichlorvos treatment presumably result from direct alkylation of DNA (Bridges et al., 1973; Green et al., 1973, 1974a,b). In the standard *E. coli* DNA polymerase-deficient assay system, dichlorvos (6.4 mmol/litre) gave a positive result (Rosenkranz, 1973; Rosenkranz & Leifer, 1980). In measuring mutation to tryphophan independence in *E. coli* strain WP2, it was found that 5 mg dichlorvos/litre was mutagenic in this test system (Green et al., 1976). Griffin & Hall (1978) have found that dichlorvos (1 mg/ml) causes breaks in colicinogenic plasmid E1 DNA from *E. coli*. In a rec-type repair test with *Proteus mirabilis* strains PG 713 (rec^-hcr^-) and PG 273 (wild type), dichlorvos (10 or 40 μmol per plate) induced base-pair substitutions and other DNA damage. In the same test, desmethyldichlorvos, at the same concentrations, gave negative results (Adler et al., 1976; Braun et al., 1982).

(b) *Mammalian cells*

In cultured V79 Chinese hamster cells, no induction of 8-azaguanine-resistant mutations after treatment with up to 1 mmol/litre dichlorvos (Wild, 1975), or of ouabain-resistant mutations after treatment with 1.25 - 5 mmol/litre dichlorvos, was found (Aquilina et al., 1984).

DNA strand breakage in cultured V79 Chinese hamster cells caused by up to 0.2% v/v dichlorvos has been reported by Green et al. (1974a). Dichlorvos (1 μl) decreased the sedimentation coefficient of calf thymus DNA upon thermal denaturation, indicating a decrease in the DNA molecular size (Rosenkranz & Rosenkranz, 1972). Incubation of dichlorvos (45 mmol/litre) with calf thymus DNA did not result in changes in thermal melting curves or DNA fractionation on a hydroxyapatite column. However, changes were observed by means of differential pulse polarography, indicating that single-stranded segments and thermolabile regions were formed in the DNA. This behaviour could perhaps be a consequence of guanine alkylation followed by depurination and chain cutting at elevated temperatures (Olinski et al., 1980).

The resistance of methylated DNA in Chinese hamster ovary cells, labelled with ^{14}C-thymidine and methyl-^{3}H-1-methionine, to micrococcal nuclease digestion was abolished when the cells were treated with dichlorvos (10 mmol/litre) for 3 h. No effects were observed on kinetics of total DNA digestion. These results indicate a conformational change in chromatin induced by dichlorvos (Nishio & Uyeki, 1982).

Dichlorvos (0.03 and 0.1 mmol/litre) has been found to induce sister chromatid exchanges (SCEs) in cultures of Chinese hamster ovary cells (Nishio & Uyeki, 1981). On the other hand, in Chinese hamster V79 cells (clone number 15), SCEs were not induced by 0.1 mmol dichlorvos/litre, but only by 0.2 and 0.5 mmol/litre solutions. The number of polyploid cells was increased at both 0.1 and 5 mmol/litre (Tezuka et al., 1980).

Dichlorvos has been tested in two independent laboratories for its ability to increase the transformation of Syrian hamster embryo cells by simian adenovirus SA_7. Pre-treatment of hamster cells with dichlorvos at concentrations of 0.05 up to 0.45 mmol/litre produced a significant enhancement of SA_7 transformation at 0.11 mmol/litre and higher (Hatch et al., 1986).

The mouse peripheral blood lymphocyte (PB) culture system has also been used to test for SCE induction. Male B6C3F1 mice were injected intraperitoneally with 5, 15, 25, or 35 mg dichlorvos/kg body weight, but there was no change in the baseline SCE frequency (Kligerman et al., 1985).

Dichlorvos (6.5 - 650 mmol/litre) has been found to induce dose-dependent unscheduled DNA synthesis in the human epithelial-like cell line EUE (Benigni & Dogliotti, 1980a,b; Aquilina et al., 1984). Both scheduled and unscheduled DNA synthesis of human lymphocytes showed dose-related inhibition by dichlorvos (5 -500 mg/litre), as measured by ^{3}H-thymidine uptake (Perocco & Fini, 1980).

Dichlorvos (0.0001 - 0.1 mmol/litre) does not induce DNA repair in human kidney T-cells. This was shown by a lack of dichlorvos-induced ^{3}H-thymidine incorporation into T-cells in the G1- or G2-phase of the cell cycle. No induction of single-strand breaks in the T-cell DNA, as measured by alkaline sucrose gradients, was found following treatment for 1, 2, or 4 h with 0.0001 - 1 mmol dichlorvos/litre (Bootsma et al., 1971).

No clear effect on the frequency of SCEs in human lymphocytes or human fetal lung fibroblasts was found after exposure to 2.5 - 10 mg dichlorvos/litre for 72 h (Nicholas et al., 1978).

In studies by Dean (1972b), human blood samples were treated with dichlorvos (0.0001 - 1 mmol/litre) for 1, 2, 4, and 20 h, after which the lymphocytes were stimulated to divide using phyto-haemagglutinin. The toxic effect of 1 mmol dichlorvos/litre was indicated by a decreased mitotic index. Mitotic cells were analysed for chromosome aberrations, but the number of dicentrics in dichlorvos-treated cells was no different from that found in untreated cells (Bootsma et al., 1971). When dichlorvos (1 - 40 mg/litre) was added at specific intervals to cultures of human lymphocytes, cytotoxicity was found at 5 mg/litre or more, but no chromosome aberrations (chromatid gaps or breaks) were detected (Dean, 1972b).

Negative results in cultured human lymphocytes were also reported by Fahrig (1974) and Wild (1975).

8.6.2.2 In vivo studies

(a) *Drosophila melanogaster*

Negative results were obtained in the standard Muller-5 test for sex-linked lethal mutations and in the induced crossing-over test with the approximate LD_{50} concentration (0.035% dichlorvos) (Jayasuriya & Ratnayake, 1973). Similarly, 0.0006 - 0.6 μmol dichlorvos gave negative results in the standard Muller-5 test (Sobels & Todd, 1979).

In studies by Hanna & Dyer (1975), a *Drosophila melanogaster* population was continuously exposed to gradually increasing concentrations of dichlorvos (because of development of increased resistance) in the food medium (up to 0.75 mg/kg food) for about 18 months. At the end of this period, an increased accumulation of mutations was observed.

Gupta & Singh (1974) reported studies where female *D. melanogaster* flies were kept on food with 1 - 50 mg dichlorvos (Nuvan 100 EC)/kg. No eggs were laid at 10 mg/kg or more, and at 1 mg/kg, survival of the eggs was 45% of that of the controls. Salivary gland chromosome abnormalities were observed in fully-grown larvae fed 1 mg/kg. However, Kramers & Knaap (1978), using the same route of administration, found no induction of sex-linked recessive lethals by dichlorvos (0.009, 0.048, and 0.09 mg/kg food).

(b) *Host-mediated assays*

Dichlorvos was not mutagenic in host-mediated assays in NMRI mice using:

(i) *S. typhimurium* (G46 his$^-$) and *Serratia marcescens* (a 21 leu$^-$) after an intraperitoneal injection of 25 mg dichlorvos/kg body weight (Buselmaier et al., 1972, 1973);

(ii) *S. typhimurium* (64-320) after an oral dose of 0.2 mg per animal (equivalent to 8 - 10 mg/kg body weight) (Voogd et al., 1972); or

(iii) *Saccharomyces cerevisae* (D4 ade2 and trp_5 loci) after an oral dose of 50 or 100 mg/kg body weight (or after exposure of CF1 mice for 5 h to 60 or 90 mg dichlorvos/m^3) (Dean et al., 1972).

Although dichlorvos was mutagenic to *S. cerevisae* in *in vitro* studies, these *in vivo* studies proved to be negative.

(c) *Dominant lethal assays*

Negative results were reported in a test for dominant lethal mutations in ICR/Ha mice (expressed as an increase in early fetal deaths or, indirectly, by pre-implantation losses), after a single intraperitoneal injection of 13 or 16.5 mg/kg body weight or five consecutive daily oral doses of 5 or 10 mg/kg body weight. The total mating period was 8 weeks (Epstein et al., 1972). The same result was obtained after exposure of male CF1 mice to 30 or 55 mg/m^3 for 16 h or to 2.1 or 5.8 mg/m^3 for 23 h daily for 4 weeks (Dean & Thorpe, 1972b).

A statistically significant increase in the frequency of pre-implantation losses in mice (Q strain) in the second week and fifth week of mating has been observed after a single intraperitoneal

Dahmen et al., 1981).

In studies by Degraeve et al. (1982, 1984a), male Q strain mice received drinking-water with 2 mg dichlorvos/litre (equivalent to 0.32 mg/kg body weight per day) 5 days per week, for 7 consecutive weeks. At the end of this period, the males were mated for 1 week with untreated virgin females, and the pregnant females were killed 14 days after the start of pregnancy. No dominant lethal mutations were induced. The same result was obtained when female CF1 mice were either given single oral doses of 0, 25, or 50 mg dichlorvos/kg body weight or continuously exposed to atmospheres containing 0, 2, or 8 mg dichlorvos/m^3 from weaning until 11 weeks of age. They were either mated at the end of the dosing or inhalation period or at intervals of 5, 10, and 15 days thereafter (Dean & Blair, 1976).

(d) *Chromosome abnormalities*

Male Q strain mice receiving drinking-water containing 2 mg dichlorvos/litre (equivalent to 0.32 mg/kg body weight), 5 days per week for 7 weeks, did not show chromosome damage in bone marrow cells, spermatogonia, or primary spermatocytes (Moutschen-Dahmen et al., 1981; Degraeve et al., 1982, 1984a); neither did mice of the same strain given a single intraperitoneal injection with 10 mg/kg body weight (Moutschen-Dahmen et al., 1981; Degraeve et al., 1984b).

In a micronucleus test, Swiss mice were given daily intraperitoneal injections of dichlorvos (0.0075 - 0.015 mg/kg body weight per day) for 2 days and killed 6 h after the last dose. No induction of aberrations in the structure or number of chromosomes in bone marrow cells was observed (Paik & Lee, 1977).

CF1 mice exposed to concentrations of 64-72 mg dichlorvos/m^3 for 16 h or to 5 mg/m^3 per day, 23 h per day, for 21 days, did not show chromosome abnormalities in bone marrow or spermatocytes. Similar results for Chinese hamsters exposed by the inhalation route to 28 -36 mg/m^3 for 16 h (males only), or by a single oral dose of 15 mg/kg body weight (males) or 10 mg/kg body weight (females), have been reported (Dean & Thorpe, 1972a).

Dichlorvos has been tested for its ability to induce *in vivo* chromosomal aberrations in Syrian hamsters bone marrow cells. Four dose levels (3, 6, 15, and 30 mg/kg body weight) were given intraperitoneally. Statistically significant increases in the number of cells with aberrant chromosomes (mainly breaks and gaps) were observed (Dzwonkowska & Hübner, 1986).

8.7 Carcinogenicity

8.7.1 Oral

8.7.1.1 Mouse

Carcinogenicity studies were carried out on two groups of 50 male and 50 female B6C3F1 mice fed 1000 and 2000 mg dichlorvos (94%) in corn oil/kg diet for 80 weeks. Due to severe signs of intoxication, doses were lowered after 2 weeks to 300 and 600 mg/kg for the remaining 78 weeks. Samples of the diets analysed during the study showed dichlorvos contents within 5% of the intended concentrations. Matched controls consisted of 10 mice of each sex; the pooled controls consisted of 100 male and 80 female mice. All surviving mice were killed at 92 - 94 weeks. Hair loss and rough hair coats were noted in many treated animals, particularly in the male groups, beginning at week 20 and persisting throughout the study. The average body weights of the high-dose mice of both sexes were slightly decreased compared with controls. The low-dose female group showed the poorest survival; 74% of the animals lived to 90 weeks. There was no significant increase in the incidence of tumours attributable to dichlorvos in either sex, i.e., dichlorvos was not demonstrated to be carcinogenic (NCI, 1977; Weisburger, 1982).

In other studies, groups of 50 male and 50 female B6C3Fl mice, 6 weeks of age, were given drinking-water with 0, 400, or 800 mg dichlorvos/litre *ad libitum*. The drinking-water solutions were renewed daily. All surviving animals were killed during week 102. A dose-dependent inhibition of body weight increase was observed throughout the study in both sexes at both dichlorvos concentrations. There was no adverse effect on mortality. The survival rates at week 102 were 62%, 66%, and 84% in males (in controls, low-, and high-dose groups, respectively), and 66%, 50%, and 80% in females. The corresponding figures for tumour incidence were 22.4%, 39.1%, and 23.4% in males and 29.3%, 16.2%, and 9.1% in females. The main tumours that were found were lung adenomas and tumours in the liver, spleen, thymus, and salivary gland. These tumours occurred in all three groups. There was no statistically significant difference in the incidence of tumours at any site in any group (Konishi et al., 1981).

Preliminary results are available from a recently completed 2-year mouse carcinogenicity study using dichlorvos. Groups of 50 male and 50 female B6C3Fl mice were given dichlorvos (dissolved in corn oil) by oral gavage daily for 2 years. Dose levels for male mice were 0, 10, or 20 mg/kg body weight per day and for female mice 0, 20, or 40 mg/kg. There were no statistically significant differences in survival rates between the treated and control male mice, and the same applied to female mice. A statistically significant increase in the incidence of forestomach squamous cell papillomas was observed in the female mice receiving 40 mg/kg per day. Two forestomach squamous cell carcinomas were also seen in this group, but none were observed in the controls or the 20 mg/kg group. Considerably fewer forestomach squamous cell papillomas were observed in male mice. Nevertheless, a non-significant increase was observed in the 20 mg/kg per day group. No forestomach squamous cell carcinomas were noted in any male group. Forestomach hyperplasia occurred relatively frequently in both control and treated male and female mice, the incidence being similar in all groups (NTP, 1987).

8.7.1.2 Rat

In studies reported by NCI (1977) and Weisburger (1982), two groups each of 50 male and 50 female Osborne-Mendel rats were fed either 150 or 1000 mg dichlorvos (94%) in corn oil/kg diet for 80 weeks. Due to the severe signs of intoxication, the 1000 mg/kg dose was reduced to 300 mg/kg diet after 3 weeks for the remaining 77 weeks. The diets were stored under conditions designed to minimize loss of dichlorvos, and the animals received fresh diets daily. Matched controls comprised 10 rats of each sex; the pooled controls consisted of 60 rats of each sex. The surviving rats were killed after 110 weeks. The average body weights of the rats receiving the high dose level were slightly decreased compared with controls. There was no significant increase in the incidence and type of tumours in either sex as a result of dichlorvos treatment.

Enomoto et al. (1981) carried out studies on groups of 50 male and 50 female Fisher 344 rats, 6 weeks of age, given drinking-water (renewed daily) containing 0, 140, or 280 mg dichlorvos/litre *ad libitum*. All surviving animals were killed in week 108 (104 weeks of exposure followed by a 4-week recovery). Slight inhibition of body weight increase was observed in males in the high-dose group, but there was no influence on mortality. The survival rates in week 108 were 82%, 75%, and 75% in males and 86%, 71%, and 82% in females, respectively, in control, low-dose, and high-dose groups. A great number of organs and tissues were selected for microscopy. The organs and tissues of all animals which died or which were killed in moribund conditions were microscopically examined, as were all tumours and macroscopical lesions. A number of animals with no specific changes were also examined. The overall tumour incidences were 100%, 96%, and 98% in males and 37%, 31%, and 33% in females, respectively, in control, low-dose, and high-dose groups. High incidences of interstitial cell tumours of the testes in males (49/51, 41/48, and 47/48, respectively) were observed in all three groups. Mononuclear cell leukaemia was found in all groups at 4 - 12%. There was no statistically significant difference in tumour incidence at any site in any group.

Preliminary results are available from a recently completed 2-year rat carcinogenicity study using dichlorvos. Dichlorvos, dissolved in corn oil, was administered each day by oral gavage to groups of 50 male and 50 female Fischer 344 rats at dose levels of 0, 4, or 8 mg/kg body weight per day. Though survival rates were slightly decreased in the treated male and female groups compared with those of their respective controls groups, the differences were not statistically significant. However, a statistically-significant and dose-related increase in the incidence of pancreatic adenomas was observed in the male rats fed 4 or 8 mg/kg. In female rats fed 8 mg/kg, a non-significant increase in pancreatic adenomas was observed. There was a relatively high incidence of pancreatic hyperplasia and atrophy in all groups of male rats, including the controls, and a lower incidence in all female groups. A statistically significant (but not dose-related) increased incidence of mononuclear leukaemia was observed in the male rats fed 4 or 8 mg/kg. A similar incidence was observed in all female groups, including the control group. Since this is a common and variable systemic lesion in Fischer-344 rats, the toxicological significance of this finding is uncertain. It is possible that its incidence in the male control group was unusually low. An increased incidence of mammary gland fibroadenomas (not dose related) was observed in the treated female rats, but these were not considered to be of toxicological concern. In addition, mammary gland hyperplasia was frequently observed in all control and treated female groups at similar incidences (NTP, 1986).

As reported in section 8.4.1.1, Witherup (1967, 1971) found no increase in tumour incidence following dichlorvos treatment of rats.

8.7.2 Inhalation

8.7.2.1 Rat

In the studies by Blair et al. (1976) described in section 8.4.2.1, no dose-related increase in tumour incidence was found.

8.7.3 Appraisal of carcinogenicity

The majority of the mouse and rat studies using dichlorvos are considered to be negative regarding carcinogenic potential (Witherup et al., 1967, 1971; Blair et al., 1976; NCI, 1977; Enomoto et al., 1981; Konishi et al., 1981; Weisburger, 1982). However, preliminary information from two recent studies on the mouse and rat, respectively, has provided equivocal evidence of carcinogenicity (NTP, 1986)[a].

The increased incidence of forestomach tumours in the mouse study is likely to be related to the route of administration (oral gavage), which has been shown in other mouse studies to induce forestomach tumours due to repeated and direct irritation of the gastric mucosa. If so, ingestion of food by human beings could not result in such

---

[a] The NTP Peer Review Panel reviewed these studies and came to the following conclusions:

"Under the conditions of these 2-year gavage studies, there was some evidence of carcinogenic activity of dichlorvos for male F344/N rats, as shown by increased incidences of adenomas of the exocrine pancreas and mononuclear cell leukemia. There was equivocal evidence of carcinogenic activity of dichlorvos for female F344/N rats, as shown by increased incidence of adenomas of the exocrine pancreas and mammary gland fibroadenomas. There was some evidence of carcinogenic activity of dichlorvos for male B6C3F1 mice and clear evidence for female B6C3F1 mice, as shown by increased incidences of forestomach squamous cell papillomas" (NTP, 1988).

direct effects on the stomach wall. Furthermore, human beings do not possess a stomach wall comparable with the forestomach of the mouse, except perhaps for the oesophagus. However, the transient passage of food through the oesophagus would probably not allow sufficient time for the carcinogenic event to occur.

Similarly, the pancreatic adenomas observed in the NTP rat study may be related to the corn oil used in the study. Evidence from other rat studies in which corn oil was used as a vehicle suggests that this is a possibility. On the other hand, it does not explain why a higher incidence of pancreatic tumours was observed in the treated animals compared with the controls. Although increased incidences of mononuclear leukaemia were observed in treated male rats, the incidence in the control group of this common and variable tumour may have been low. The evidence for carcinogenicity in these two recent studies is difficult to interpret at present. When complete and final reports of these studies become available, more definitive conclusions may be drawn.

8.8 Mechanisms of Toxicity; Mode of Action

A full description of the mechanism of action can be found in Environmental Health Criteria 63: Organophosphorus Insecticides - A General Introduction (WHO, 1986b).

Dichlorvos directly inhibits AChE activity in the nervous system and other tissues. This reaction takes place in three steps:

(a) reversible binding of dichlorvos to the enzyme;

(b) reaction with the enzyme to form a dimethylphospho-enzyme derivative, with the loss of DCA; and

(c) "aging" of the phospho-enzyme compound to a more stable methylphospho-enzyme derivative.

Reaction (a) is rapid, but reversible. Reaction (b) is also rapid, but the phosphorylated enzyme can be returned to its native state spontaneously only by hydrolysis at very slow rates or by agents such as *N*-methyl 2-pyridinium aldoxime (2-PAM) at higher rates. Reaction (c) is comparatively slow ($t_{\frac{1}{2}}$ = about 2.5 h at 37 °C and pH 7.4), but the product has the same stability as that of erythrocytes ($t_{\frac{1}{2}}$ = about 120 days) (Gillett et al., 1972).

Death due to poisoning is caused by excessive cholinergic effects such as bronchospasms, hypersecretion from cholinergic innervated glands (especially critical in lungs and bronchi), and cardiac disturbances caused by vagotonus and anoxia. Convulsions and paralysis in skeletal musculature are caused by brain anoxia as well as cholinergic effects within the central nervous system.

In vivo studies on the inhibition of ChE activity resulting from a single oral or parenteral dose of dichlorvos, at various time intervals, after dosing are summarized in Table 18. In general, the maximum inhibition occurred within 1 h, and was followed by rapid recovery. Dogs seemed to be more sensitive than rats, and showed a slower recovery.

Dichlorvos, when infused intravenously (into the ear vein) of adult male rabbits, produced dose- and time-related inhibition of whole blood ChE activity during infusion. Spontaneous but incomplete recovery to 60 - 80% of the normal activity occurred within 60 - 90 min of infusion (Shellenberger et al., 1965; Gough & Shellenberger, 1970, 1977-78; Shellenberger, 1980).

In a study on the influence of temperature on ChE activity, rats were injected intraperitoneally with a single dose of 6.25 mg dichlorvos (95%)/kg and kept at either 28 °C or 5 °C. The maximum inhibition of whole blood ChE activity (40%) occurred after 0.5 h. The animals at 5 °C showed less inhibition and a faster recovery of whole blood ChE activity than those at 28 °C (Chattopadhyay et al., 1982).

8.9 Neurotoxicity

8.9.1 Delayed neurotoxicity

A detailed description of the neurotoxic potential of organophosphorus compounds can be found in Environmental Health Criteria 63: Organophosphorus Insecticides - A General Introduction (WHO, 1986b).

Several studies have shown that dichlorvos does not produce delayed neurotoxicity in pre-medicated hens, whether it is administered orally or subcutaneously (Durham et al., 1956; Aldridge & Barnes, 1966; Johnson, 1969, 1975a,b, 1978, 1981; Aldridge & Johnson, 1971; Lotti & Johnson, 1978). The inhibition of brain neurotoxic esterase (NTE) without signs of ataxia has been observed (Aldridge & Johnson, 1971; Johnson, 1978).

Caroldi & Lotti (1981) reported mild signs of ataxia in pre-medicated hens 2 weeks after a single massive subcutaneous dose (100 mg/kg body weight) and severe inhibition of NTE in peripheral nerve, spinal cord, and brain. However, Johnson (1978) did not observe ataxia in pre-medicated hens given the same dose in the same way. These hens showed severe inhibition of brain NTE but far less inhibition of spinal cord NTE. It appears that ataxia arises from the inhibition of spinal cord NTE. When the dose was repeated 1 - 3 days after the first dose, spinal cord NTE inhibition increased and the hens became ataxic.

White leghorn hens have been used in a 90-day study on the neurotoxic potential of dichlorvos (99.9%) after dermal or oral administration. For oral administration, a 10 - 20% solution of dichlorvos in corn oil in gelatin capsules was used whereas, dermally, 1 - 20% emulsifiable concentrates in technical grade xylene (containing 2% Triton X-100) were used. Dichlorvos at doses greater than 1 mg/kg

Table 18. Time-related ChE activity in animals after administration of a single dose of dichlorvos

Species/sex	Route	Dose (mg/kg body weight)	Time	Cholinesterase activity (%)			Reference
				plasma	erythrocyte	brain	
Mouse (male)	intraperitoneal	30	15 min			37	Cohen & Ehrich (1976)
			2 h			40	
			5 h			69	
			18 h			92	
Mouse (male)	intraperitoneal	10	15 min			30	Nordgren et al. (1978)
			60 min			50	
			2 h			80	
Rat (male)	oral	50	15 min	30	20	10-15	Modak et al. (1975)
			3 h	30	65		
			24 h	60	75	60-70	
Rat (male)	oral	40	1 h			30	Teichert et al. (1976)
Rat (male)	oral	40	5 min			55	Pachecka et al. (1977)
			15 min			20	
			2 h			30	
			24 h			75	
			48 h			100	
Rat (male)	intravenous	2.5	30 min	40		15	Reiner & Plestina (1979)
			90 min	60		35	
			3 h	90		55	
			12 h	100		80	
			48 h			90	
Dog (beagle) (sex not specified)	oral	50	2 h	32	63		Ward & Glicksberg (1971)
			24 h	63	74		
			5 days	92	78		
			21 days	100	92		
Dog (greyhounds and crossbred)	oral	22	1 h	12	17		Snow & Watson (1973)
			3 h	24	34		
			24 h	70	65		
			72 h	95	65		

body weight per day (dermal) or 6 mg/kg (oral) led to cholinergic symptoms including salivation, convulsions, and death after 2 - 3 days. With oral doses of 3 - 6 mg/kg no ataxia or death was observed. Dermally, dichlorvos was very toxic for hens. Dose levels of about 1.7 and 3.3 mg/kg for an average period of 37 days caused ataxia and death. An average dermal dose level of 0.65 mg/kg body weight for 90 days did not induce ataxia or death. Typical symptoms of organophosphorus-ester-induced delayed neurotoxicity (OPIDN) were not observed (Francis et al., 1985).

In summary, it is possible to produce clinical neuropathy in hens, but the doses required are far in excess of the LD_{50}. The effects are associated with severe inhibition of NTE in brain and spinal cord, measured shortly after dosing (Johnson, 1981).

8.9.2 Mechanism of neurotoxicity

Male rats given a lethal intraperitoneal injection of 40 mg dichlorvos/kg body weight did not show electrocortical disturbances. Deaths resulted from respiratory failure (Hyde et al., 1978).

In studies by Desi (1983), adult CFY rats were given daily oral doses ranging from 1.25 to 4 mg dichlorvos/kg body weight mixed in the diet for 3 months. Plasma, erythrocyte, and brain ChE activities were comparable with those of control rats. Increased EEG activity and enhanced central excitability were found in the male rats only.

No changes in reflex motor unit potential activity or in nerve conduction velocity were noted in dogs 7 days after single oral doses of 30, 59.5, or 148 mg dichlorvos/kg body weight. However, erythrocyte ChE activity was inhibited at all doses, and the highest dose produced signs of intoxication (Hazelwood et al., 1979).

A single oral dose of 40 mg dichlorvos/kg or repeated doses of 1.6 mg/kg body weight per day did not cause histological abnormalities in the brain of adult Wistar rats. Repeated administration of 50% of the LD_{50} (i.e., 40 mg/kg body weight per day for 10 - 21 days), caused myelin pallor and micro-vacuolation of the white matter. It seems likely that primary degeneration of axons and secondary myelin sheath abnormalities caused the spongy tissue loosening observed under the electron microscope (Zelman, 1977; Zelman & Majdecki, 1979).

In studies by Ali et al. (1979a) and Hasan et al. (1979), male rats were given 3 mg dichlorvos/kg per day intraperitoneally for 10 days. Following perfusion-fixation, sections of cerebellum and spinal cord were studied with the electron microscope. An abnormal increase in the number of mitochondria in the spinal cord was found. Myelin degeneration was detected in the spinal cord and myelin figures were occasionally noted within oedematous dendrite profiles.

Another study of dichlorvos neurotoxicity involved the investigation of lipid peroxidation. This entails the direct reaction between oxygen and lipids to form free-radical intermediates and semi-stable peroxides. Major cellular components, such as membranes and subcellular organelles, are damaged by these free radicals. Hasan &

Ali (1980) found a dose-dependent increase in the rate of lipid peroxidation in various regions of the brain of the rat after intraperitoneal administration of dichlorvos (at concentrations ranging from 0.6 to 3 mg/kg body weight, daily) for 10 days. Also, there was an increased incidence of lipofuscin-like pigment in the Purkinje cells of the cerebellar cortex.

Maslinska et al. (1984) found that dichlorvos (dose levels of 4 - 8 mg/kg body weight for 10 days) affected the phospholipid-protein balance in the brain of rabbits. The animals were exposed during the postnatal "critical" life period, which constitutes a turning point in the development of the brain. At this time, the neurons have already undergone considerable arborization, and myelination and vascularization are expanding rapidly. In addition, the overall oxygen consumption is reaching its steepest rate of increase. In the myelin sheaths under formation, several phospholipids are deposited. The authors found changes in the phospholipid-protein ratio which correlated well with the observed delay in myelin sheath formation. Ultrastructural changes in certain subcellular organelles may be connected with the change in this ratio, since it is crucial to the structural and functional properties of the membranes and enzymes bound to them.

Dambska et al. (1984) have studied the influence of dichlorvos on blood vessel walls, the perivascular area, and the permeability of the blood-brain barrier in young rabbits. The young animals received 9 mg dichlorvos/kg body weight for 16 days starting on the 6th day of life. There was a decrease in ChE activity in brain capillary walls. Electron microscopic studies showed lesions of the perivascular astrocytes and changes in the endothelial cells. However, these lesions did not disturb the blood-brain barrier mechanism for horseradish peroxidase particles.

Studies on the central cholinergic system have revealed that the inhibition of brain ChE activity and its subsequent recovery were uniform in all brain regions studied in orally dosed (50 mg/kg) rats. ACh concentrations were increased in brain areas within 15 min of treatment. A biphasic effect was observed on choline metabolism in the brain. The cortex was more cholinergic than the striatum in terms of percentage increase in ACh and choline (Modak et al., 1975). In a similar study on rats, either receiving a single oral dose (40 mg/kg) or repeated oral doses (4 mg/kg), the activity of whole brain choline acetyltransferase and the contents of ACh and choline in whole brain were not altered, though brain ChE activity was markedly inhibited. However, in the cerebral hemispheres, and especially the corpus striatum, the ACh level was considerably increased, without a concomitant change in choline (Teichert et al., 1976).

Kobayashi et al. (1980, 1986) investigated the concentration of total, free, labile-bound and stable-bound ACh in the brain of rats given single or multiple subcutaneous injections of dichlorvos (0.2 - 4 mg/kg body weight). The results suggest that alterations in the mobilization and storage of ACh in the central cholinergic nerves may be induced. The time course for ACh accumulation was measured in rat brain regions after intravenous treatment with 15 mg dichlorvos/kg body weight (Stavinoha et al., 1976). The striatum had the highest rate of accumulation and the cerebellum the lowest. The calculated turnover time for the different regions of the brain was between 0.9 and 5.6 min.

In studies by Ali & Hasan (1977) and Ali et al. (1979b, 1980), rats were given intraperitoneally 3 mg dichlorvos/kg body weight per day for 10 or 15 days. The concentrations of dopamine, norepinephrine, and 5-hydroxytryptamine (5-HT) were significantly decreased in different parts of the brain, and 5-HT was significantly increased in the spinal cord.

A single dose or short-term (12 weeks) treatment of rats with high concentrations of dichlorvos, which produced brain ChE inhibition, resulted in decreased norepinephrine levels in the brain (Brzezinski & Wysocka-Paruszewska, 1980). From these studies, it was suggested that the metabolism of catecholamines and 5-HT may be disturbed by dichlorvos.

8.10 Other Studies

Many studies in different organ systems have been carried out. In most of these studies, the route of administration was the oral or intraperitoneal route. Single or repeated dosing was used, mainly with high dose levels, in mice and rats. The influence on brain enzymes (other than brain ChE), liver enzymes such as ChE (inhibition), microsomal cytochrome P-450 activity (decrease), drug-metabolizing enzyme activity, and UDP-glucuronyl transferase (no influence), and many other enzyme systems were studied.

Furthermore, the influence of dichlorvos on adrenal steroidogenesis has been investigated (Civen et al., 1980).

8.10.1 Immunosuppressive action

A dose-related suppression of the humoral immune response induced by *S. typhimurium* was observed in rabbits orally administered 0.3 - 2.5 mg dichlorvos (93%)/kg body weight in capsules, 5 times a week for 6 weeks (Desi et al., 1978).

In a comparable study on rabbits, the cellular immune response was estimated using the tuberculin skin test. The skin redness in the tuberculin test and the serum antibody titres of treated animals showed a dose-dependent decrease compared with those of controls (Desi et al., 1980).

8.11 Factors Modifying Toxicity; Toxicity of Metabolites

8.11.1 Factors modifying toxicity

In studies on the effect of diet on the toxicity of dichlorvos, young male rats were kept for 30 days on the following synthetic diets:

high protein (HPD), low protein (LPD), high fat (HFD), and standard (SD). Growth rates were normal except for a slightly decreased body weight gain in the HFD group. The composition of the diet, *per se*, did not significantly affect plasma and erythrocyte ChE activity 24 h or 5 days after dosing. A single intraperitoneal injection of 50 mg dichlorvos/kg body weight led to higher mortality in LPD rats (as expected with a protein-deficient diet) and lower mortality in HPD rats, compared with SD animals (Purshottam & Kaveeshwar, 1979).

In a further study, growing male rats were kept on an HFD or HPD for 30 days. At the end of this period, a single intraperitoneal dose of dichlorvos (20 or 30 mg/kg body weight) was administered. Results showed that diets, *per se*, did not affect initial plasma or erythrocyte ChE activity, nor did the HPD or HFD diets protect against mortality from dichlorvos. In the case of the HPD, the spontaneous recovery of ChE activity was reduced in the plasma and erythrocytes of dichlorvos-treated rats. However, with an HFD, this recovery was significantly increased (Purshottam & Srivastava, 1984).

Costa & Murphy (1984) studied the interaction between acetaminophen (which, like dichlorvos, is detoxified by glutathione transferase) and dichlorvos (10 mg/kg body weight) in mice. Acetaminophen (600 mg/kg body weight) pre-treatment did not have any affect on dichlorvos toxicity. On the other hand, intraperitoneal pre-treatment with diethylmaleate (1 ml/kg body weight) increased the acute toxicity of dichlorvos.

8.11.2 Toxicity of metabolites

8.11.2.1 Acute toxicity

The toxicity of metabolites of dichlorvos in female mice, injected intraperitoneally, is considerably less than that of dichlorvos (Table 19).

Mice (male and female) survived a single exposure of 130 mg DCA/m^3 for 5 - 7 h (Stevenson & Blair, 1969).

8.11.2.2 Short-term exposures

Groups of 20 male and 20 female rats were exposed for 30 days to actual concentrations of 0 or 0.5 - 1 mg DCA/m^3. Half the animals were then killed promptly and the remainder on day 35. After 30 days of exposure, the male rats showed a slight decrease in body weight and food intake, and a slight increase in absolute and relative liver weight. There were no such changes in the rats left for 5 more days unexposed to DCA. Histological examination of the lungs of exposed males and females revealed a higher incidence of minor inflammatory changes than in controls. No other changes attributable to DCA were found in general health, behaviour, haematology, clinical chemistry, organ weights, gross pathology, or histopathology. A similar study using groups of 10 male and 10 female rats and actual concentrations of

Table 19. Intraperitoneal LD_{50} values of metabolites of dichlorvos in female mice[a]

Compound	Vehicle	LD_{50} (mg/kg body weight)
desmethyldichlorvos, sodium salt	water	1500
dichloroacetyaldehyde (DCA)	corn oil	440
dichloroethanol	corn oil	890
dichloroacetic acid	corn oil or water	250
sodium dichloroacetate	water	3000
methyl and dimethyl phosphoric acid mixture	water	1500
sodium methyl- and dimethylphosphate mixture	water	3000

[a] From: Casida et al. (1962).

0 or approximately 2 mg/m³ DCA revealed no abnormalities attributable to DCA (Wilson & Dix, 1973).

8.11.2.3 Long-term exposure

No long-term tests have been carried out with DCA as such. However, in the 2-year oral studies on rats and dogs with dichlorvos (section 8.4.1), the degradation product DCA was present in the test diets in increasing amounts, so that possible effects of DCA were included in the results of these studies.

8.11.2.4 Mutagenicity

DCA appears to be mutagenic in the *Salmonella* test using *S. typhimurium* TA100. The mutagenicity decreased in the presence of a microsomal activation system. Part of the decrease was dependent on the presence of the co-factors NADP and glucose-6-phosphate. No evidence for mutagenicity with 2,2-dichloroethanol was obtained in this *S. typhimurium* strain (Löfroth, 1978).

In a dominant lethal assay, a single intraperitoneal injection of 176 mg DCA/kg in male mice (AB Jena-Halle strain) produced a decrease in the number of total implants and live fetuses in the first 3 weeks of the test, and an increase in post-implantation losses. The same test was repeated with a strain of mice (DBA) less sensitive to mutagenic effects. The same effects were found, but to a lesser extent, and mainly in the fourth week (Fischer et al., 1977).

8.11.2.5 Metabolism

When ^{32}P-dimethylphosphate (500 mg/kg in water) was administered orally to a male rat, the autopsy (90 h after treatment) indicated that almost the entire dose had been eliminated. The urine, containing only unmetabolized dimethylphosphate, accounted for about half of the radioactivity. The tissues were almost devoid of ^{32}P-containing material (Casida et al., 1962).

A rat, orally dosed with 500 mg/kg ^{32}P-desmethyldichlorvos in water, excreted about 14% of the dose in the urine in 90 h. The tissue distribution of ^{32}P was similar to that which followed ^{32}P-dichlorvos administration. The very high proportion of radioactivity in the bone was indicative of rapid degradation to phosphoric acid (Casida et al., 1962).

9. EFFECTS ON MAN

9.1 General Population Exposure

9.1.1 Acute toxicity

9.1.1.1 Poisoning incidents

A 56-year-old woman ingested an estimated amount of 100 mg dichlorvos/kg body weight and survived, following intensive care for 14 days (Watanabe et al., 1976). However, a suicide with a dichlorvos dose of about 400 mg/kg succeeded in spite of treatment (Shinoda et al., 1972).

A 35-year-old female patient accidently ingested 60 g fluid Divipan (dichlorvos concentration not reported). She was comatose for one week and recovered slowly. Clinical and electrophysiological examinations (no details reported) showed a pure motor form of neuropathy, according to the authors (Vasilescu & Florescu, 1980).

Two cases of poisoning with dichlorvos taken orally in unspecified, but high, quantities have been reported. The patients first showed signs of severe anti-ChE poisoning. After recovery, delayed neurotoxicity developed. They showed a severe axonal degeneration neuropathy. One of them recovered within 12 months (Wadia et al., 1985).

Reeves et al. (1981) reported six cases, over an 8-year period, of bone-marrow failure (pancytopenia) in children shortly after exposure to dichlorvos and propoxur. Van Raalte & Jansen (1981) doubted the causal relationship between dichlorvos and bone-marrow failure in the children, because the disease has not been observed in workers with high exposure, or in the general population. In addition, haematotoxic effects have not been observed in experimental animals.

9.1.2 Effects of short- and long-term exposure

In the 1960s, field studies were carried out in several countries to test dichlorvos as a residual insecticide for malaria control in houses. Numerous residents of all ages and conditions were exposed without any adverse effects attributable to dichlorvos being reported (Escudié & Sales, 1963; Funckes et al., 1963; Gratz et al., 1963; Quarterman et al., 1963; Foll et al., 1965). In two field studies, the plasma and erythrocyte ChE activities were measured in adults and young children. No abnormalities were found, though air concentrations of dichlorvos in the treated houses rose to 0.8 mg/m^3 (Funckes et al., 1963; Gratz et al., 1963).

In a report by Gold et al. (1984), 20 single-family residences were treated with a 0.5% solution of dichlorvos (at an average rate of 0.189 g/m^2) to control the cockroach *Blattella germanica* L. The average air concentration for the first 2 h after treatment was

548 μg/m^3 and for the next 2 h was 183 μg/m^3. Pesticide operators and the residents of treated structures were monitored for evidence of dichlorvos exposure, using exposure pads, air samples, serum and erythrocyte ChE tests, and urinalyses. There was no evidence of dichlorvos or dichloroacetic acid in urine. There were slight, but statistically significant, changes in the mean serum ChE activity of some of the residents of treated structures, but the mean erythrocyte ChE was unchanged.

Passengers in an aircraft provided with an automatic insect-control system, which released 0.15 - 0.30 mg dichlorvos/m^3 for periods of about 30 min, did not show any signs of discomfort (Jensen et al., 1965). Tests have shown that man can withstand daily exposure to concentrations of 0.5 mg/m^3 without clinical effects, and with only a slight depression of blood ChE activity (Hayes, 1961). Three men exposed to approximately the same level during 24 tests did not show any change in blood ChE activity (Schoof et al., 1961).

A case of chronic obstructive bronchitis ascribed to exposure to dichlorvos was described by Barthel (1983). However, it could not be excluded that other components of the unknown formulation could have been the cause. ChE determinations were not performed.

9.1.2.1 Studies on volunteers

Single oral doses (1 - 32 mg/kg body weight) of dichlorvos in a slow-release PVC formulation administered to 107 male volunteers produced measurable reductions in erythrocyte ChE activity at dose levels above 4 mg/kg, with a maximum reduction of 46% at the highest dose. Plasma ChE activity was affected at lower doses, with 50% reduction at 1 mg/kg and about 80% at 6 mg/kg or more. Repeated oral doses of 1 - 16 mg/kg body weight per day were given to 38 volunteers for up to 3 weeks. The plasma ChE activity was maximally depressed at all dose levels, and the erythrocyte ChE activity depression was dose related and significant at 2 mg/kg or more. Blood cell count, urine, liver function, prothrombin time, and blood urea nitrogen were all normal (Hine & Slomka, 1968, 1970; Slomka & Hine, 1981).

In studies by Rider et al. (1968), dichlorvos was given to groups of five men at daily oral doses of 1, 1.5, 2, or 2.5 mg per man. The plasma ChE activity of the 2.5 mg group was reduced by 30% after 20 days of treatment. Administration of 2 mg for 28 days resulted in a reduction of 30% 2 days after the last dose. Erythrocyte ChE activity was not significantly affected in either group (Rider et al., 1967). Daily oral doses of 1.5 mg per man given to 10 volunteers for 60 days caused a significant reduction (approximately 40%) in plasma ChE activity, which returned to normal levels when dichlorvos administration was discontinued.

Boyer et al. (1977) reported studies on two groups of six men (21 - 45 years of age) who received 0.9 mg of dichlorvos three times a day for 21 days. One group received the dichlorvos in a gelatin salad, the other in a pre-meal capsule filled with cottonseed oil. Two other groups of six men received placebo treatment. No consistent cholinomimetic signs or symptoms were observed, nor was erythrocyte ChE inhibited. However, plasma ChE was significantly depressed within 20 days, although the extent depended on the method by which dichlorvos was administered. Recovery was comparable in both groups, the half-life for the regeneration of plasma ChE being 13.7 days.

Volunteers did not show inhibition of plasma or erythrocyte ChE activity either when handling a dichlorvos strip for 30 min each day or after having a piece of the strip applied to the arm for 30 min each day for 5 consecutive days (Zavon & Kindel, 1966).

The wearing of dichlorvos-impregnated garments by babies for 48 - 84 h did not produce changes in either plasma or erythrocyte ChE activity over a period of 5 days (Cavagna et al., 1969).

In studies on eight volunteers, carried out in an aircraft at operational cabin altitude (2400 m), no changes in plasma or erythrocyte ChE activity, dark adaptation, or bronchiolar resistance were observed. Dichlorvos concentration in the air ranged from 0.73 to 1.18 mg/m^3 during exposures of 45 min (Smith et al., 1972).

Hunter (1970a) reported studies on 26 men (21 - 57 years of age) and 6 women (19 - 25 years of age) who were exposed in a chamber for 2-7½ h to actual dichlorvos concentrations of approximately 1 mg/m^3. Food and drink were served in the chamber. No clinical signs were observed, and no effects on haematology, urinalysis, kidney function, EEG, ECG, respiratory activities, or erythrocyte ChE activity were found. Plasma ChE activities were markedly inhibited only when the exposure lasted over 6 - 7 h (Hunter, 1970a).

In studies by Hunter (1969, 1970b), seven men (25 - 56 years of age) were exposed (head and neck) to dichlorvos vapour (actual concentrations of 1 - 52 mg/m^3), and 6 men were exposed (head exposure only) to 7 - 50 mg/m^3, for periods from 10 min to 4 h. The maximum dose level was 52 mg/m^3 (for 65 min), and the maximum period was 240 min (at 13 mg/m^3). Symptoms were confined to irritation of the throat, some rhinorrhoea, and substernal discomfort at the highest concentrations. No effects on the pupil or on visual acuity were recorded. Erythrocyte ChE activity was depressed in only one person. However, there was a direct relationship between the reduction in plasma ChE activity and the dichlorvos dose (concentration•time). No changes were found in either kidney or pulmonary function or in the overall metabolic rate.

When three men were exposed to dichlorvos (actual concentrations of 0.3 - 0.9 mg/m^3 (mean, 0.5 mg/m^3) or 0.9 - 3.5 mg/m^3 (mean, 2.1 mg/m^3) for 1 or 2 h per day for 4 consecutive days, plasma ChE alone decreased slightly in the men exposed for 2 h per day to the higher concentration (Witter et al., 1961).

A group of 15 men (23 - 61 years of age) was exposed for up to 6 half-hour intervals per night for 14 days (total of 39 doses) to actual dichlorvos concentrations ranging from 0.14 to 0.33 mg/m^3. No clear changes in plasma ChE activity or other parameters such as reaction time, airway resistance, or vision were found. The same results were obtained when a similar group was exposed to actual concentrations of 0.1 - 0.6 mg/m^3 for intervals of 8 - 10 h, 4 nights per week for 11 weeks (Rasmussen et al., 1963).

No significant effect on plasma or erythrocyte ChE activity was observed in 14 persons exposed at the recommended rate of one dichlorvos strip per 30 m^3 in their homes over a period of 6 months. The strips were replaced at much shorter intervals than normally recommended. The air concentration 40 days after the installation of the fourth strip was approximately 0.09 mg/m^3 (Zavon & Kindel, 1966).

In three home studies involving 26 families, conducted in Arizona, USA, no deleterious effects on health or plasma or erythrocyte ChE activity were observed in the residents exposed to dichlorvos strips all over the house (8 - 10 strips) for over a year. Even monthly replacement of the strips resulted in only a slight inhibition of plasma ChE activity. The maximum air concentrations of dichlorvos averaged 0.13 mg/m^3 (Leary et al., 1971, 1974).

9.1.2.2 Hospitalized patients

In a report by Pena Chavarra et al. (1969), a single oral dose of 6 or 12 mg dichlorvos/kg body weight was administered in the form of a slow-release granular resin formulation as an anthelminthicum to 108 hospitalized adult patients, many of these debilitated and with severe anaemia. Plasma ChE activity was markedly reduced, in some patients by 76 - 100%. However, erythrocyte ChE activity was much less inhibited. No symptoms of intoxication were observed, except for brief mild headaches in a few patients, and there were no abnormalities in haematological studies or in hepatic and renal function tests.

In studies by Cervoni et al. (1969), single doses of dichlorvos (PVC-resin formulations) were administered orally 2 h before breakfast to 705 adults found to be harbouring infections of *Trichuris*, hookworm, or *Ascaris*. Six or 12 mg dichlorvos/kg body weight resulted in infection cure rates of approximately 70 - 100%. According to the authors, minimum to modest plasma ChE depression and zero to minimum erythrocyte ChE depression occurred at both dose levels. No clinical symptoms or alterations in haematology or in liver and kidney function were observed.

Sick adults and children and healthy pregnant women and babies in hospital wards treated with dichlorvos strips (one strip per 30 or 40 m^3) had normal erythrocyte ChE activities. Only subjects exposed for 24 h per day to dichlorvos concentrations above 0.1 mg/m^3 or patients with liver insufficiency showed even a moderate decrease in plasma ChE activity (Cavagna et al., 1969, 1970; Cavagna & Vigliani, 1970).

9.2 Occupational Exposure

9.2.1 Acute toxicity

9.2.1.1 Poisoning incidents

A number of fatal and non-fatal poisoning cases have been described after concentrated formulations of dichlorvos splashed onto parts of the body. Two workers who failed to wash it off promptly died consequently. However, in those cases where the spilled solution was washed off immediately, the victims showed symptoms of intoxication but recovered after treatment. A serious non-fatal case occurred after a spillage of 120 ml of a 3% formulation that was not washed off immediately. After 1½ h, the victim developed slurred speech, became drowsy, and collapsed. He recovered completely after treatment (Hayes, 1963, 1982).

A pest-control operator became contaminated with a 1% solution of dichlorvos in mineral spirit after using a leaking knapsack sprayer. The man changed his overalls and completed his day's work. He noticed weakness, dizziness, and difficulty in breathing. Contact dermatitis developed on the back skin. After the fourth day, his blood ChE was 36% of normal, but there were no signs of systemic illness. He recovered without medication, and the ChE activity increased to 72% of normal within one month. The acute dermatitis was probably caused by the solvent (Bisby & Simpson, 1975).

A driver of a truck transporting a 5% commercial formulation of dichlorvos (15% petroleum distillate and 80% trichloroethane) developed persistent contact dermatitis for 2 months following accidental skin contact. In addition, the patient experienced headache, mild rhinorrhoea, burning of the tongue, and a bitter taste in his mouth. Initial blood ChE levels were in the low normal range returning to the high normal range within 2 weeks. Patch tests with 1% and 0.1% dichlorvos in petroleum distillate were negative (Mathias, 1983). In view of the symptoms and the slight ChE inhibition, it seems likely that trichloroethane caused the dermatitis.

Cronce & Alden (1968) described four people who handled dogs wearing anti-flea dog collars containing 9 - 10% dichlorvos. Acute primary contact dermatitis was described. Closed patch tests with 0.25, 0.5, and 1% dichlorvos in distilled water and in mineral oil were positive in all four people. General experience with the collars indicates that only a few people are susceptible to this kind of irritation (Hayes, 1982).

9.2.2 Effects of short- and long-term exposure

9.2.2.1 Pesticide operators and factory workers

The effect on sprayers of dichlorvos fume, used inside a building for cockroach control, was examined. When 0.3 - 0.6% dichlorvos oil spray was used at the rate of 6 ml/m^2 by the sprayers (7 - 9 people), inhibition of ChE activity in the subjects was 15%, and conjunctival injections or sore throats were observed in some sprayers after either 18 min or 4 h of spraying operation. To examine the effect of elevated dichlorvos vapour pressure at higher temperatures, four men sprayed 0.6% oil spray for 2 h at the room temperature of 25 °C. The inhibition of plasma and erythrocyte ChE activities was 22% and 7%, respectively. In another study, 11 sprayers used 0.6% oil spray for 6 h of actual work time at 20 °C without rest. Two of them showed an inhibition of plasma ChE activity of 38% while the others did not show significant inhibition of erythrocyte ChE. It was concluded that conjunctival injections and sore throats were attributable to the kerosene solvent used and that the 38% depression in ChE activity was probably due to long hours of continuous work. Therefore, the overall effect on ChE activity was not considered to be severe (Ueda et al., 1959, 1960).

Twelve fogging machine operators did not show any reduction in plasma or erythrocyte ChE activity when applying 4% dichlorvos aerosols in tobacco warehouses for 16 h per week, over a period of 2 - 4 months (Witter, 1960).

Sixteen men replacing old dichlorvos dispensers and installing new units in houses in Haiti, 5 days per week for 3 weeks, showed a decrease of up to 60% in plasma ChE activity. No signs or symptoms of intoxication were observed. Air concentrations ranged from 0.3 to 2.1 mg/m^3 (Stein et al., 1966).

The blood ChE activity of sprayers, exposed during insect control in grain stores to air concentrations of 1.9 - 3 mg/m^3 dichlorvos, was reduced to 19 - 23% (Sasinovich, 1970).

In a report by Das et al. (1983), each of 13 pesticide-control operators carried out urban pest-control for one day in four houses using 230 - 330 g dichlorvos as aerosol and 40 - 50 g dichlorvos as emulsion spray. At the end of the day's work, an operator had an average dichlorvos residue of 0.8 mg/m^2 on the back, 0.4 mg/m^2 on the chest, and 11 mg/m^2 on the respirator filter. Dimethylphosphate was detected in the urine, but blood and urine analyses, including serum ChE levels, did not reveal any other changes in clinical parameters.

In the course of either the production or processing of a dichlorvos-releasing product, 11 male and 2 female factory workers were exposed to an average dichlorvos concentration of 0.7 mg/m^3 (highest value 3 mg/m^3) on each working day for a period of 8 months. Inhibition of plasma ChE activity was noted within a few days of the start of exposure, while inhibition of erythrocyte ChE activity developed much more slowly. The maximum plasma ChE activities recorded were 40% lower than the pre-exposure levels, but 60% lower than the post-exposure levels. Erythrocyte ChE activity was reduced by approximately 35% compared with pre- and post-exposure levels. One month after exposure had ceased, plasma ChE and erythrocyte ChE activities were found to have returned to normal physiological levels.

The other haematological investigations and the medical examinations did not reveal any changes attributable to dichlorvos exposure (Menz et al., 1974).

9.2.2.2 Mixed exposure

A number of articles have described the symptoms found in individual workers or groups of workers exposed for a number of years to different types of pesticides, including dichlorvos. In general, a slight-to-moderate decrease in ChE activity occurred. Furthermore, several complaints and symptoms were noticed, but no clear clinical poisoning cases occurred. These case studies are, however, of little relevance for the evaluation of dichlorvos because of the mixed exposure to different pesticides (Bellin & Chow, 1974; Fournier et al., 1976; Gupta et al., 1979; Ullmann et al., 1979; Hayes et al., 1980; Hayes, 1982).

From 1975 to 1977, 88 patients with pesticide dermatitis, 15 suffering from photo-dermatitis, were studied. Patch tests using 29 different pesticides of different categories were carried out, but did not lead to an identification of the responsible pesticides. Eight out of 52 patients (15.4%) reacted positively to a photopatch (Horiuchi & Ando, 1978; Horiuchi et al., 1978).

Stoermer (1985) described a case of contact dermatitis in a woman who had worked as a pest controller for 3 months and had sprayed dichlorvos and propoxur. She was treated and recovered within one week.

A field survey of tea growers was made in the Chiran area of Japan in 1982. Out of 84 tea growers examined (21 men and 63 women), 5 women had contact dermatitis from agricultural work. Dichlorvos was among the insecticides, fungicides, and herbicides used. Patch tests showed relatively high rates of positive reactions with dichlorvos (27% of women and 5% of men). Also, cross-sensitization was found between methidathion and dichlorvos (Fujita, 1985).

10. EVALUATION OF HUMAN HEALTH RISKS AND EFFECTS ON THE ENVIRONMENT

10.1 Evaluation of Human Health Risks

Since 1961, dichlorvos, an organophosphate with anti-ChE activity, has been used worldwide as a contact and stomach insecticide to control insects on crops and domestic animals. It is also used as an insecticide in houses and other buildings and for insect control in aircraft.

Dichlorvos is readily absorbed by the body of mammals through all routes of exposure, and is readily metabolized in the liver. Within 1 h of oral administration, dichlorvos is found in the liver, kidneys, and other organs of experimental animals. It is rapidly eliminated via the kidneys, with a half-life of 14 min.

The metabolism of dichlorvos in various species, including human beings, follows similar pathways. Differences between species relate only to the *rate* of metabolism, but this is always rapid.

Dichlorvos is moderately to highly toxic for mammals (the oral LD_{50} for the rat is 30 - 110 mg/kg body weight). The classification of dichlorvos by WHO (1986a) is based on an oral LD_{50} for the rat of 56 mg/kg body weight. Signs of intoxication usually occur shortly after exposure and are typical of an organophosphorus pesticide. Inhibition of ChE activity is a sensitive criterion of exposure. In short-term toxicity studies on mammals, it was shown that ChE activity was not decreased at oral dose levels below about 0.5 mg/kg body weight. In long-term studies on rats at oral dose levels of 2.5 mg/kg body weight or more, hepatocellular fatty vacuolization was seen. At 0.25 mg/kg body weight, no ChE inhibition was found, nor were there any other effects.

Reproduction and teratogenicity studies using a wide range of dose levels (6.25 - 500 mg/kg body weight) were negative. Dichlorvos showed alkylating properties in *in vitro* but not in *in vivo* studies. Many *in vitro* mutagenicity studies with bacteria and yeast were positive, while the *in vivo* studies were mainly negative. From the available mutagenicity studies, it is unlikely that dichlorvos constitutes a mutagenic hazard for man. Carcinogenicity studies on mice and rats fed dichlorvos (dose levels of up to 234 mg/kg diet) were negative. Two recent carcinogenicity studies have been carried out on mice and rats in which dichlorvos was administered by intubation for up to 2 years at dose levels of 10 - 40 mg/kg body weight (mice) and 4 or 8 mg/kg body weight (rats). Only preliminary information has been provided. The evidence for carcinogenicity in these new studies is difficult to interpret at this time. Only when complete and final reports become available will it be possible to draw more definite conclusions (in this context, see footnote p 95, section 8.7.3).

From work on hens, the suspicion of delayed neurotoxicity from dichlorvos has neither been established nor totally refuted. However, there have been two clinical reports on four patients suffering intense poisoning from dichlorvos taken orally who survived with treatment and who then displayed neurotoxic effects. Thus, the possibility of delayed neurotoxicity in man cannot be entirely discounted, but it is likely to occur only with excessive oral doses.

Human volunteers who were given single or repeated oral doses of 2 mg/kg body weight or more showed significant inhibition of erythrocyte ChE activity. At 1 mg/kg body weight, no such inhibition was found.

The application of dichlorvos to crops and animals results in residues that rapidly disappear by volatilization and hydrolysis. In general, residues of dichlorvos and the breakdown product DCA in food commodities are low and will be further reduced during processing. The exposure of the general population to dichlorvos by food and drinking-water is negligible, as is confirmed in total-diet studies.

In short-term inhalation studies on mammals, 1 or 2 mg dichlorvos/m^3 did not inhibit ChE activity.

In a 2-year, 23 h/day, whole-body inhalation study on rats, 0.48 mg/m^3 caused inhibition of plasma and erythrocyte activity, but brain AChE activity was not inhibited and there were no clinical signs. An unquantified, but considerable, extra exposure, resulting from the grooming of contaminated fur and contamination of food and drinking-water, had contributed to this effect. The no-observed-adverse-effect level was 0.05 mg/m^3. There was no evidence of carcinogenicity.

In a 6- to 7-h exposure of human volunteers to approximately 1 mg dichlorvos/m^3, only plasma ChE activity was inhibited. The erythrocyte AChE activity, taken to be representative of the AChE activity in the nervous tissue, was unaffected.

Residents exposed for over one year to an average air concentration of 0.1 mg/m^3 arising from slow-release strips showed no inhibition of plasma or erythrocyte ChE activity and no deleterious effects on health.

The main exposure of the general population is by inhaling dichlorvos when used indoors to control insects. The recommended use (one slow-release strip/ 30 m^3) will give concentrations in the air of up to 0.1 - 0.3 mg/m^3 in the first few days, decreasing thereafter to below 0.1 mg/m^3. The air concentration depends on temperature, humidity, and ventilation.

As long as approved slow-release strips are used according to the label instructions, no health hazard can be expected for man. However, special care may need to be taken with young children and sick or elderly people who are especially vulnerable when continuously exposed (24 h per day) in poorly ventilated rooms. Other methods of indoor application should be equally safe if the label instructions are followed.

There is some indication that dichlorvos may induce dermatitis and cross-sensitization in people handling various types of pesticides including dichlorvos.

In occupational conditions, the main route of exposure to organophosphorus pesticides is usually the dermal route. In the case of dichlorvos, with its high vapour pressure, exposure by inhalation is also important. In these occupational situations, the dichlorvos concentrations in the air are generally below 1 mg/m^3 but, in certain circumstances, they may rise considerably above this level. This stresses the need for adequate protective measures to be taken during occupational exposure and regular monitoring of ChE activity.

10.2 Evaluation of Effects on the Environment

The presence of dichlorvos in the environment as a result of accidental losses or direct application on soil or in water will not lead to long-term effects because of its fast breakdown and evaporation. Furthermore, it is converted to a number of compounds, such as dichloroacetic acid, by microorganisms. Certain bacteria species can use dichlorvos as a sole carbon source, while others cannot and are inhibited in their growth. Therefore, its influence on microorganisms is complex.

Dichlorvos is moderately to highly toxic (range, 0.2 - 10 mg/litre) for freshwater and estuarine species of fish and invertebrates. In certain fish, concentrations of 0.25 - 1.25 mg/litre cause inhibition of brain and liver ChE activity. Concentrations of as little as 0.05 mg/litre may have deleterious effects, particularly in invertebrates. Dichlorvos has a high toxicity for birds and bees. Caution is advised in the use and handling of dichlorvos where these species might be exposed.

No bioaccumulation occurs in the different environmental compartments and organisms.

10.3 Conclusions

1. Exposure of the general population to dichlorvos via food and drinking-water is negligible and does not constitute a health hazard.

2. The in-house use of dichlorvos as an insecticide in the form of sprays or slow-release strips (at recommended levels) does not constitute a short- or long-term hazard for the general population. However, continuous (24 h per day) exposure of young children and diseased or elderly people in non-ventilated or poorly ventilated rooms should be avoided.

3. In spite of their toxicity, dichlorvos and its formulations do not contribute an undue hazard to those occupationally exposed, provided that adequate ventilation and skin protection are used.

4. Except under conditions of gross spillage, the recommended use of dichlorvos as an insecticide does not constitute an acute or long-term hazard for aquatic or terrestrial organisms, although there may be an acute hazard for birds and bees.

11. RECOMMENDATIONS

1. Continuous (24 h/day) exposure of young children and diseased or elderly people to dichlorvos in non-ventilated or poorly ventilated rooms should be avoided.

2. As dichlorvos from different sources may vary in purity and type of impurities, attention should be paid to its composition. This should conform to FAO and WHO specifications (FAO, 1977; WHO, 1985). In the case of formulations, potential hazards of other components, such as solvents and stabilizers, should also be considered.

12. PREVIOUS EVALUATIONS BY INTERNATIONAL BODIES

Dichlorvos was evaluated by the Joint FAO/WHO Meeting on Pesticide Residues (JMPR) in 1965, 1966, 1967, 1969, 1970, 1974, and 1977 (FAO/WHO, 1965a,b, 1967a,b, 1968a,b, 1970a,b, 1971a,b, 1975a,b, 1978a,b). In 1966, the JMPR established an Acceptable Daily Intake (ADI) for human beings of 0 - 0.004 mg/kg body weight, which remains unchanged.

The Pesticide Development and Safe Use Unit, Division of Vector Biology and Control, WHO, has classified technical dichlorvos as "highly hazardous" (Class IB) (Plestina, 1984; WHO, 1986a) and has produced a safety sheet on dichlorvos (No. 75.2) (WHO/FAO, 1975-86).

Specifications for dichlorvos use in public health and in plant protection have been published by WHO (1985) and FAO (1977), respectively.

In 1979, the International Agency for Research on Cancer (IARC) came to the following conclusions in considering the carcinogenicity of dichlorvos:

(a) dichlorvos was tested in different animal species via different routes; no conclusive evaluation on the basis of these studies could be made;

(b dichlorvos is an alkylating agent and binds to bacterial and mammalian nucleic acids;

(c) it is a mutagen in a number of microbial systems, but there is no evidence of its mutagenicity in mammals, in which it is rapidly degraded.

In the evaluation by IARC, it was stated that "the available data do not allow an evaluation of the carcinogenicity of dichlorvos to be made".

In its series "Scientific Reviews of Soviet Literature on Toxicity and Hazards of Chemicals", the International Register of Potentially Toxic Chemicals has published a volume on dichlorvos (IRPTC, 1984).

REFERENCES

ABBOTT, D.C., CRISP, S., TARRANT, K.R., & TATTON, J.O.G. (1970) Pesticide residues in the total diet in England and Wales. III. Organophosphorus pesticide residues in the total diet, 1966-67. *Pestic. Sci.*, **1**: 10-13.

ACKERMAN, H., LEXOW, B., & PLEWKA, E. (1969) [Detection and identification of the organic phosphate, phosphorothionate, phosphonate, and carbamate insecticides in biological material.] *Arch. Toxicol.*, **24**: 316-324 (in German).

ADLER, B., BRAUN, R., SCHONEICH, J., & BOHME, H. (1976) Repair-defective mutants of *Proteus mirabilis* as a prescreening system for the detection of potential carcinogens. *Biol. Zentralbl.*, **95**: 463-469.

ALABASTER, J.S. (1969) Survival of fish in 164 herbicides, insecticides, fungicides wetting agents and miscellaneous substances. *Int. pest Control*, **11**(2): 25-35.

ALDRIDGE, W.N. & BARNES, J.M. (1966) Further observations on the neurotoxicity of organophosphorus compounds. *Biochem. Pharmacol.*, **15**: 541-548.

ALDRIDGE, W.N. & JOHNSON, M.K. (1971) Side effects of organophosphorus compounds: delayed neurotoxicity. *Bull. World Health Organ.*, **44**: 259-263.

ALDRIDGE, W.N. & JOHNSON, M.K. (1977) Mechanisms and structure-activity relationships providing a high safety factor for anti-cholinesterase insecticides. In: *Proceedings of the 1977 British Crop Protection Conference - Pests and Diseases, Croyden, British Crop Protection Council*. pp. 721-729.

ALI, M.S., RAHMATULLAH, M., JAHAN, R., YUSUF, H.K.M., & CHOWDHURY, A.A. (1979c) Effect of DDVP (insecticide) on citric acid fermentation in *Aspergillus niger*. *Enzyme Microb. Technol.*, **1**: 127-128.

ALI, S.F. & HASAN, M. (1977) Effect of organophosphate insecticide dichlorvos on the amino acid content of different regions of the rat brain and spinal cord. *Indian J. exp. Biol.*, **15**(9): 759-761.

ALI, S.F., HASAN, M., & MITRA, S.C. (1979a) Organophosphate DDVP-induced changes in the rat spinal cord: an electron microscopic and biochemical study. *J. Anat. Soc. India*, **28**(1): 36.

ALI, S.F., HASAN, M., & TARIQ, M. (1979b) Levels of dopamine, norepinephrine, and 5-hydroxytryptamine in different regions of rat brain and spinal cord following chronic administration of organophosphate pesticide dichlorvos. *Indian J. exp. Biol.*, **17**(4): 424-426.

ALI, S.F., CHANDRA, O., & HASAN, M. (1980) Effects of an organophosphate (dichlorvos) on open-field behaviour and locomotor activity: correlation with regional brain monoamine levels. *Psychopharmacology*, **68**(1): 37-42.

ALLEN, S.D., VANKAMPEN, K.R., & BROOKS, D.R. (1978) Evaluation of the feline dichlorvos (DDVP) flea collar. *Feline Pract.*, **8**(3): 9-16.

AMBRUS, A., LANTOS, J., VISI, E., CSATLOS, I., & SARVARI, L. (1981) General method for determination of pesticide residues in samples of plant origin, soil, and water. *J. Assoc. Off. Anal. Chem.*, **64**(3): 733-768.

ANDERSON, R.A., BARSTAD, J.A.B., & LAAKE, K. (1978) An improvement of the spectrophotometric method for determination of cholinesterase activity in erythrocytes and tissue homogenates. *Ann. Natl Inst. Publ. Health (Norway)*, **1**(1): 51-55.

ANON. (1972) Vapona insecticide. In: *Analytical methods for pesticides and plant growth regulators*, Modesto, California, Shell Development Company, **Vol. 6**, pp. 529-541.

ANON. (1973) The determination of malathion and dichlorvos residues in grain. Report by the Panel on Malathion and Dichlorvos Residues in Grain. *Analyst*, **98**: 19-24.

ANON. (1977) Determination of residues of organophosphorus pesticides in fruits and vegetables. Report by the Panel on Determination of Residues of Certain Organophosphorus Pesticides in Fruits and Vegetables. *Analyst*, **102**: 858-868.

ANON. (1982) *Pesticides: a safety guide*, London, Shell International Chemical Company Ltd, pp. 53-55.

AOKI, Y., TAKEDA, M., & UCHIYAMA, M. (1975) Comparative study of methods for the extraction of eleven organophosphorus pesticide residues in rice. *J. Assoc. Off. Agric. Chem.*, **58**(6): 1286-1293.

AQUILINA, G., BENIGNI, R., BIGNAMI, M., CALCAGNILE, A., DOGLIOTTI, E., FALCONE, E., & CARERE, A. (1984) Genotoxic activity of dichlorvos, trichlorfon, and dichloroacetaldehyde. *Pestic. Sci.*, **15**: 439-442.

ARATAKE, Y. & KAYAMURA, T. (1973) [Toxicity of insecticides to silkworm larvae.] *Sanshi Kenkyu (Acta serol.),* **87**: 68-78 (in Japanese).

ARIMATSU, S., HOSHIRO, Y., & NOMURA, T. (1977) [Studies on primary irritation test of pesticides in rabbits.] *Nippon Noson Igakkai Zasshi,* **26**: 572-573 (in Japanese).

ASHWOOD-SMITH, M.J., TREVINO, J., & RING, R. (1972) Mutagenicity of dichlorvos. *Nature (Lond.),* **240**: 418-420.

ATKINS, E.L., GREYWOOD, E.A., & MACDONALD, R.L. (1973) *Toxicity of pesticides and other agricultural chemicals to honey bees,* Riverside, University of California (Agricultural Extension Report No. M-16 Rev. 9/73).

AUGUSTINSSON, K.B., ERIKSSON, H., & FAIJERSSON, Y. (1978) A new approach to determining cholinesterase activities in samples of whole blood. *Clin. Chim. Acta,* **89**: 239-252.

AULICINO, F., BIGNAMI, M., CARERE, A., CONTI, G., MORPURGO, G., & VELCICH, A. (1976) Mutational studies with some pesticides in *Aspergillus nidulans. Mutat. Res.,* **38**(2): 138.

BAKSI, S.N. (1978) Effect of dichlorvos on embryonal and fetal development in thyro-parathyroidectomized thyroxine-treated and euthyroid rats. *Toxicol. Lett.,* **2**(4): 213-216.

BALLINGTON, P.E., SKIPPER, H.D., & HEGG, R.O. (1978) Response of coliform populations in poultry waste digesters to three insecticides. *J. environ. Qual.,* **7**(2): 262-264.

BARTHEL, E. (1983) [Irritative and allergic effects of pesticide aerosols on the respiratory tract and problems of their evaluation.] *Z. gesamte Hyg.,* **29**(11): 678-681 (in German).

BATORA, V., VITOROVIC, S.L.J., THIER, H.P., & KLISENKO, M.A. (1981) Development and evaluation of simplified approaches to residue analysis. *Pure appl. Chem.,* **53**: 1039-1049.

BATTE, E.G., ROBINSON, O.W., & MONCOL, D.J. (1969) Influence of dichlorvos on swine reproduction and performance of offspring to weaning. *J. Am. Vet. Med. Assoc.,* **154**(11): 1397.

BAZER, F.W., ROBSON, O.W., & ULBERG, L.C. (1969) Effect of dichlorvos and PMS on reproduction in swine. *J. anim. Sci.,* **28**: 145.

BEDFORD, C.T. & ROBINSON, J. (1972) The alkylating properties of organophosphates. *Xenobiotica,* **2**(4): 307-337.

BELL, TH.G., FARRELL, K., PADGET, G.A., & LEENDERTSEN, L.W. (1975) Ataxia, depression, and dermatitis associated with the use of dichlorvos-impregnated collars in the laboratory cat. *J. Am. Vet. Med. Assoc.*, **167**(7): 575-586.

BELLIN, J.S. & CHOW, I. (1974) Biochemical effects of chronic low-level exposure to pesticides. *Res. Commun. chem. Pathol. Pharmacol.*, **9**(2): 325-337.

BENIGNI, R. & DOGLIOTTI, E. (1980a) UDS studies on selected environmental chemicals. *Mutat. Res.*, **74**: 248-249.

BENIGNI, R. & DOGLIOTTI, E. (1980b) UDS studies on selected environmental chemicals. *Mutat. Res.*, **74**(3): 217.

BENIGNI, R., BIGNAMI, M., CAMONI, I., CARERE, A., CONTI, G., IACHETTA, R., MORPURGO, G., & ORTALI, V.A. (1979) A new *in vitro* method for testing plant metabolism in mutagenicity studies. *J. Toxicol. environ. Health*, **5**: 809-819.

BERAN, F. (1970) [Present knowledge on the toxicity of our pesticides to bees.] *Gesunde Pflanz.*, **22**(2): 21-31 (in German).

BIGNAMI, M., CONTI, L., MORPURGO, G., & VELCICH, A. (1976) Comparative analysis of different test systems for somatic recombination with *Aspergillus nidulans*. *Mutat. Res.*, **38**(2): 138-139.

BIGNAMI, M., AULICINO, F., VELCICH, A., CARERE, A., & MORPURGO, G. (1977) Mutagenic and recombinogenic action of pesticides in *Aspergillus nidulans*. *Mutat. Res.*, **46**: 395-402.

BISBY, J.A. & SIMPSON, G.R. (1975) An unusual presentation of systemic organophosphate poisoning. *Med. J. Aust.*, **2**: 394-395.

BLAIR, D. & RODERICK, H.R. (1976) An improved method for the determination of urinary dimethyl phosphate. *J. agric. food Chem.*, **24**(6): 1211-1223.

BLAIR, D., HOADLEY, E.C., & HUTSON, D.H. (1975) The distribution of dichlorvos in the tissues of mammals after its inhalation or intravenous administration. *Toxicol. appl. Pharmacol.*, **31**: 243-253.

BLAIR, D., DIX, K.M., HUNT, P.F., THORPE, E., STEVENSON, D.E., & WALKER, A.I.T. (1976) Dichlorvos: a 2-year inhalation carcinogenesis study in rats. *Arch. Toxicol.*, **35**: 281-294.

BOOTSMA, D., HEERING, H., KLEIJER, W.J., BUDKE, L., DE JONG, L.P.A., & BERENDS, F. (1971) *Effects of dichlorvos on human cells in tissue culture. A progress report*, Rijswijk, The Netherlands, Medical Biological Laboratory TNO (Report No. MBL 1971-5).

BOUSH, G.M. & MATSUMURA, F. (1967) Insecticidal degradation by *Pseudomonas melophthora*, the bacterial symbiote of the apple maggot. *J. econ. Entomol.*, **60**: 918-920.

BOWMAN, B.T. & SANS, W.W. (1983) Determination of octanol- water partitioning coefficients (K_{ow}) of 61 organophosphorus and carbamate insecticides and their relationships to respective water solubility (S) values. *J. environ. Sci. Health*, **B18**(6): 667-683.

BOYER, A.C., BROWN, L.J., SLOMKA, M.B., & HINE, C.H. (1977) Inhibition of human plasma cholinesterase by ingested dichlorvos: effect of formulation vehicle. *Toxicol. appl. Pharmacol.*, **41**: 389-394.

BRADWAY, D.E., SHAFIK, T.M., & LORES, E.M. (1977) Comparison of cholinesterase activity, residue levels, and urinary metabolite excretion of rats exposed to organophosphorus pesticides. *J. agric. food Chem.*, **25**(6): 1353-1358.

BRAUN, R., SCHONEICH, J., WEISSFLOG, L., & DEDEK, W. (1982) Activity of organophosphorus insecticides in bacterial tests for mutagenicity and DNA repair: direct alkylation vs metabolic activation and breakdown. I. Butonate, vinylbutonate, trichlorfon, dichlorvos, desmethyldichlorvos, and demethylvinyl-butonate. *Chem.-biol. Interact.*, **39**: 339-350.

BRIDGES, B.A., MOTTERSHEAD, R.P., GREEN, M.H.L., & GRAY, W.J.H. (1973) Mutagenicity of dichlorvos and methyl methanesulfonate for *Escherichia coli* WP2 and some derivatives deficient in DNA repair. *Mutat. Res.*, **19**: 295-303.

BROWN, V.K.H. & ROBERTS, M. (1966) *The anti-acetylcholinesterase activity of technical DDVP when administered percutaneously to guinea-pigs*, Sittingbourne, Shell Research Ltd (Unpublished Report No. IRR TL/40/66).

BROWN, V.K.H. & STEVENSON, D.E. (1962) *Agricultural chemicals: therapy of DDVP intoxication by atropine and cholinesterase reactivators*, Sittingbourne, Shell Research Ltd (Shell Technical Memorandum No. TOX 31/62) (Unpublished Report).

BROWN, V.K.H., BLAIR, D., HOLMES, D.L., & PICKERING, R.G. (1968) *The toxicity of low concentrations of dichlorvos by inhalation in rodent and avian species*, Sittingbourne, Shell Research Ltd (Unpublished Report No. TLGR.0015.68).

BRUNGS, W.A., MCCORMICK, J.H., NEIHEISEL, T.W., SPEHAR, R.L., STEPHAN, C.E., & STOKES, G.N. (1977) Effects of pollution on fresh-water fish. *J. Water Pollut. Control Fed.*, **49**(6): 1425-1493.

BRYANT, R.J. & MINETT, W. (1978) A gas chromatographic method for the determination of dichlorvos in air. *Pestic. Sci.*, **9**: 525-528.

BRZEZINSKI, J. & WYSOCKA-PARUSZEWSKA, B. (1980) Neurochemical alterations in rat brain as a test for studying the neurotoxicity of organophosphorus insecticides. *Arch. Toxicol.*, **4**(Suppl.): 475-478.

BULL, D.L. & RIDGWAY, R.L. (1969) Metabolism of trichlorfon in animals and plants. *J. agric. food Chem.*, **17**(4): 837-841.

BUNDING, I.M., YOUNG, R., Jr, SCHOOLEY, M.A., & COLLINS, J.A. (1972) Maternal dichlorvos effects on farrowing parameters. *J. anim. Sci.*, **35**: 238.

BUSELMAIER, W., ROHRBORN, G., & PROPPING, P. (1972) [Mutagenicity investigations with pesticides in the host-mediated assay and the dominant lethal test in mice.] *Biol. Zentralbl.*, **91**(3): 311-325 (in German).

BUSELMAIER, W., ROHRBORN, G., & PROPPING, P. (1973) Comparative investigations on the mutagenicity of pesticides in mammalian test systems. *Mutat. Res.*, **21**(1): 25-26.

BUTLER, G.L. (1977) Algae and pesticides. *Residue Rev.*, **66**: 40.

CARERE, A., CARDAMONE, G., ORTALI, V., BRUZZONE, M.L., & DI GIUSEPPE, G. (1976) Mutational studies with some pesticides in *Streptomyces coelicolor* and *Salmonella typhimurium*. *Mutat. Res.*, **38**(2): 136.

CARERE, A., ORTALI, V.A., CARDAMONE, G., TORRACCA, A.M., & RASCHETTI, R. (1978a) Microbiological mutagenicity studies of pesticides *in vitro*. *Mutat. Res.*, **57**: 277-286.

CARERE, A., ORTALI, V.A., CARDAMONE, G., & MORPURGO, G. (1978b) Mutagenicity of dichlorvos and other structurally-related pesticides in *Salmonella* and *Streptomyces*. *Chem.-biol. Interact.*, **22**: 297-308.

CAROLDI, S. & LOTTI, M. (1981) Delayed neurotoxicity caused by a single massive dose of dichlorvos to adult hens. *Toxicol. Lett.*, **9**: 157-159.

CARSON, S. (1969) *Teratology studies in rabbits (summary appraisal)*, Maspeth, New York, Food and Drug Research Laboratories (Unpublished Report, 30 June).

CARTER, M.K. & MADDUX, B. (1968) Effects of selected agents on the *in vitro* inhibition of cholinesterase activity of dichlorvos. *Pharmacologist*, **10**: 222.

CARTER, M.K. & MADDUX, B. (1974) Interaction of dichlorvos and anticholinesterases on the *in vitro* inhibition of human blood cholinesterases. *Toxicol. appl. Pharmacol.*, 27: 456-463.

CASIDA, J.E., MCBRIDE, L., & NIEDERMEIER, R.P. (1962) Metabolism of 2,2-dichlorovinyl dimethyl phosphate in relation to residues in milk and mammalian tissues. *J. agric. food Chem.*, 10(5): 370-377.

CAVAGNA, G. & VIGLIANI, E.C. (1970) Problèmes d'hygiène et de sécurité dans l'emploi du vapona comme insecticide dans les locaux domestiques. *Med. Lav.*, 61(8/9): 409-423.

CAVAGNA, G., LOCATI, G., & VIGLIANI, E.C. (1969) Clinical effects of exposure to DDVP (Vapona) insecticide in hospital wards. *Arch. environ. Health*, 19(1): 112-113.

CAVAGNA, G., LOCATI, G., & VIGLIANI, E.C. (1970) Exposure of new-born babies to Vapona insecticide. *Eur. J. Toxicol.*, 3(1): 49-57.

CERVONI, W.A., OLIVER-GONZALEZ, J., KAYE, S., & SLOMKA, M.B. (1969) Dichlorvos as a single-dose intestinal anthelmintic therapy for man. *Am. J. trop. Med. Hyg.*, 18(6): 912-919.

CHATTOPADHYAY, D.P., DIGHE, S.K., DUBE, D.K., & PURNANAND (1982) Changes in toxicity of DDVP, DFP, and parathion in rats under cold environment. *Bull. environ. Contam. Toxicol.*, 29: 605-610.

CHEN, Z.M,, ZABIK, M.J., & LEAVITT, R.A. (1984) Comparative study of thin film photodegradative rates for 36 pesticides. *Ind. eng. chem. Prod. Res. Dev.*, 23: 5-11.

CIPAC HANDBOOK (1980) *Analysis of technical and formulated pesticides*, Cambridge, Wheffer and Sons, Collaborative International Pesticides Analytical Council, Vol. 1A, pp. 1214-1224 (Addendum to CIPAC 1).

CIVEN, M., LEEB, J.E., WISHNOW, R.M., WOLFSEN, A., & MORIN, R.J. (1980) Effects of low level administration of dichlorvos on adrenocorticotrophic hormone secretion, adrenal cholesteryl ester, and steroid metabolism. *Biochem. Pharmacol.*, 29: 635-641.

CLINCH, P.G. (1970) Effect on honey bees of combs exposed to vapour from dichlorvos slow-release strips. *N.Z. J. agric. Res.*, 13(2): 448-452.

COCHRANE, W.P. (1979) Application of chemical derivatisation techniques for pesticide analysis. *J. chromatogr. Sci.*, 17: 124-137.

CODEX ALIMENTARIUS COMMISSION (1979) *Recommended method of sampling for the determination of pesticide residues. Report of the Tenth Session of the Codex Committee on Pesticide Residues,* Rome, Food and Agriculture Organization of the United Nations, Appendix IV, Annex I, pp. 67-70 (Alinorm 79/24).

CODEX ALIMENTARIUS COMMISSION (1983) *Guidelines on good analytical practice in residue analysis and recommendations for methods of analysis for pesticide residues,* Rome, Food and Agriculture Organization of the United Nations, p. 40.

COHEN, S.D. & EHRICH, M. (1976) Cholinesterase and carboxyl-esterase inhibition by dichlorvos and interactions with malathion and triorthotolyl phosphate. *Toxicol. appl. Pharmacol.,* **37**: 39-48.

COLLINS, J.A., SCHOOLEY, M.A., & SINGH, V.K. (1971) The effect of dietary dichlorvos on swine reproduction and viability of their offspring. *Toxicol. appl. Pharmacol.,* **19**: 377.

COLLINS, R.D. & DE VRIES, D.M. (1973) Air concentrations and food residues from use of Shell No-Pest[R] Insecticide Strip. *Bull. environ. Contam. Toxicol.,* **9**(4): 227-233.

COSTA, L.G. & MURPHY, S.D. (1984) Interaction between acetaminophen and organophosphate in mice. *Chem. Pathol. Pharmacol.,* **44**(3): 389-400.

COULSTON, F. & GRIFFIN, T. (1977) *Cholinesterase activity and neuromuscular functions of Rhesus monkeys exposed to DDVP vapours,* Albany, New York, Institute of Comparative and Human Toxicology and Holloman Air Force Base, International Center of Environmental Safety (Unpublished report).

CRONCE, P.C. & ALDEN, H.S. (1968) Flea-collar dermatitis. *J. Am. Med. Assoc.,* **206**(7): 1563-1564.

DALE, W.E., MILES, J.W., & WEATHERS, D.B. (1973) Measurement of residues of dichlorvos absorbed by food exposed during disinsection of aircraft. *J. agric. food Chem.,* **21**(5): 858-860.

DAMBSKA, M. & MASLINSKA, D. (1982) Effect of dichlorvos (DDVP) intoxication of rabbit brain. *Neuropathol. Pol.* **20**(1/2): 77-84.

DAMBSKA, M., MASLINSKA, D., RAKOWSKA, I., & RUTCZYNSKI, M. (1978) [Evaluation of the effect of dichlorvos poisoning of pregnant rabbits and rats on the condition and development of their offspring.] *Bromatol. Chem. Toksykol.,* **11**(3): 355-357 (in Polish).

DAMBSKA, M., IWANOWSKI, L., & KOZLOWSKI, P. (1979) The effect of transplacental intoxication with dichlorvos on the development of cerebral cortex in newborn rabbits. *Neuropathol. Pol.* **17**(4): 571-576.

DAMBSKA, M., IWANOWSKI, L., MASLINSKA, D., & OSTENDA, M. (1984) Blood-brain barrier in young rabbit brain after dichlorvos intoxication. *Neuropathol. Pol.* **22**(1): 129-137.

DARROW, D.I. (1973) Biting lice of goats: control with dichlorvos-impregnated resin neck collars. *J. econ. Entomol.*, **66**: 133-135.

DAS, Y.T., TASKAR, P.K., BROWN, H.D., & CHATTOPADHYAY, S.K. (1983) Exposure of professional pest control operator to dichlorvos (DDVP) and residue on house structures. *Toxicol. Lett.*, **17**: 95-99.

DAVIDEK, J., SEIFERT, J., & DOLEZALOVA, Z. (1976) The determination of dichlorvos in milk by using classical and square-wave polarography. *Milchwissenschaft*, **31**(5): 267-270.

DEAN, B.J. (1972a) The mutagenic effects of organophosphorus pesticides on microorganisms. *Arch. Toxikol.*, **30**: 67-74.

DEAN, B.J. (1972b) The effect of dichlorvos on cultured human lymphocytes. *Arch. Toxikol.*, **30**: 75-85.

DEAN, B.J. & BLAIR, D. (1976) Dominant lethal assay in female mice after oral dosing with dichlorvos or exposure to atmospheres containing dichlorvos. *Mutat. Res.*, **40**(1): 67-72.

DEAN, B.J. & THORPE, E. (1972a) Cytogenic studies with dichlorvos in mice and Chinese hamsters. *Arch. Toxikol.*, **30**: 39-49.

DEAN, B.J. & THORPE, E. (1972b) Studies with dichlorvos vapour in dominant lethal mutation tests on mice. *Arch. Toxikol.*, **30**: 51-59.

DEAN, B.J., DOAK, S.M.A., & FUNNELL, J. (1972) Genetic studies with dichlorvos in the host-mediated assay and in liquid medium using *Saccharomyces cerevisiae*. *Arch. Toxikol.*, **30**: 61-66.

DEDEK, W., GEORGI, W., & GRAHL, R. (1979) Comparative degradation and metabolism of ^{32}P-labelled butonate, trichlorphone and dichlorvos in crop plants. *Biochem. Physiol. Pflanz.*, **174**: 707-722.

DEGRAEVE, N., GILOT-DELHALLE, J., MOUTSCHEN, J., MOUTSCHENDAHMEN, M., COLIZZI, A., CHOLLET, M., & HOUBRECHTS, N. (1980) Comparison of the mutagenic activity of organophosphorus insecticides in mouse and in the yeast *Schizosaccharomyces pombe*. *Mutat. Res.*, **74**(3): 201-202.

DEGRAEVE, N., CHOLLET, M.C., MOUTSCHEN, J., MOUTSCHEN-DAHMEN, M., GILOT-DELHALLE, J., & COLIZZI, A. (1982) Genetic and cytogenetic effects of chronic treatment with organophosphorus insecticides. *Mutat. Res.*, **97**: 179-180.

DEGRAEVE, N., CHOLLET, M.C., & MOUTSCHEN, J. (1984a) Cytogenetic and genetic effects of subchronic treatments with organophosphorus insecticides. *Arch. Toxicol.*, **56**: 66-67.

DEGRAEVE, N., CHOLLET, M.C., & MOUTSCHEN, J. (1984b) Cytogenetic effects induced by organophosphorus pesticides in mouse spermatocytes. *Toxicol. Lett.*, **21**: 315-319.

DESI, I. (1983) Neurotoxicological investigation of pesticides in animal experiments. *Neurobehav. Toxicol. Teratol.*, **5**: 503-515.

DESI, I., VARGA, L., & FARKAS, J. (1978) Studies on the immunosuppressive effect of organochlorine and organophosphoric pesticides in subacute experiments. *J. Hyg. Epidemiol. Microbiol. Immunol.*, **22**: 115-122.

DESI, I., VARGA, L., & FARKAS, J. (1980) The effect of DDVP, an organophosphorus pesticide, on the humoral and cell-mediated immunity of rabbits. *Arch. Toxicol.*, **4**(Suppl.): 171-174.

DICOWSKY, L. & MORELLO, A. (1971) Glutathione-dependent degradation of 2,2-dichlorovinyl dimethyl phosphate (DDVP) by the rat. *Life Sci.*, **10**(2): 1031-1037.

DIKSHITH, T.S.S., DATTA, K.K., & CHANDRA, P. (1976) 90-day dermal toxicity of DDVP in male rats. *Bull. environ. Contam. Toxicol.*, **15**(5): 574-580.

DOUGHERTY, E.M., REICHELDERFER, C.F., & FAUST, R.M. (1971) Sensitivity of *Bacillus thuringiensis* var. *thuringiensis* to various insecticides and herbicides. *J. invertebr. Pathol.*, **17**: 292-293.

DMITRIEV, A.I. & KOZEMJAKJN, N.G. (1975) [Veterinary expert report on the meat of chicken poisoned by dichlorvos.] *Veterinarija*, **1975**(1): 90-92 (in Russian).

DRAGER, G. (1968) [Gas chromatographic method for the determination of dichlorvos residues in plants and milk.] *Pflanzenschutz Nachr. Bayer*, **21**(3): 377-384 (in German).

DRAUGHON, F.A. & AYRES, J.C. (1978) Effect of selected pesticides on growth and citrinin production by *Penicillium citrinum*. *J. food Sci.*, **43**: 576-578.

DURHAM, W.F., GAINES, TH.B., & HAYES, W.J. (1956) Paralytic and related effects of certain organic phosphorus compounds. *Arch. ind. Health,* **13**: 326-330.

DURHAM, W.F., GAINES, TH.B., MCCAULEY, R.H., Jr, SEDLAK, V.A., MATTSON, A.M., & HAYES, W.J., Jr (1957) Studies on the toxicity of *O,O*-dimethyl-2,2-dichlorovinyl phosphate (DDVP). *Am. Med. Assoc. Arch. Ind. Health,* **15**: 340-349.

DYER, K.F. & HANNA, P.J. (1973) Comparative mutagenic activity and toxicity of triethylphosphate and dichlorvos in bacteria and *Drosophila. Mutat. Res.,* **21**: 175-177.

DZWONKOWSKA, A. & HUBNER, H. (1986) Induction of chromosomal aberrations in the Syrian hamster by insecticides tested *in vivo. Arch. Toxicol.,* **58**: 152-156.

EDSON, E.F. (1958) Blood tests for users of organophosphorus insecticides. *World Crops,* **10 February**: 49-51.

EGYED, M.N. & BENDHEIM, U. (1977) Mass poisoning in chickens by consumption of organophosphorus (dichlorvos) contaminated drinking-water. *Refu. Vet.,* **34**(3): 107-111.

EICHNER, M. (1978) [Quick residue control of plant and animal food, tobacco, and tobacco products by Sweep-Co analysis 1.] *Z. Lebensm. Unters. Forsch.,* **167**: 245-249 (in German).

EISLER, R. (1969) Acute toxicities of insecticides to marine decapod crustaceans. *Crustaceana,* **16**: 302-310.

EISLER, R. (1970) *Acute toxicities of organochlorine and organophosphorus insecticides to estuarine fish,* Washington DC, US Department of the Interior, Fish and Wildlife Service, Bureau of Sport Fisheries and Wildlife (Technical Paper No. 46).

ELGAR, K.E. & STEER, B.D. (1972) Dichlorvos concentrations in the air of houses arising from the use of dichlorvos PVC strips. *Pestic. Sci.,* **3**: 591-600.

ELGAR, K.E., MARLOW, R.G., & MATHEWS, B.L. (1970) The determination of residues of dichlorvos in crops and tissues. *Analyst,* **95**: 875-878.

ELGAR, K.E., MATHEWS, B.L., & BOSIO, P. (1972a) Dichlorvos residues in food arising from the domestic use of dichlorvos PVC strips. *Pestic. Sci.,* **3**: 601-607.

ELGAR, K.E., MATHEWS, B.L., & BOSIO, P. (1972b) Vapona strips in shops: residues in foodstuffs. Global aspects of chemistry, toxicology, and technology as applied to the environment. *Environ. Qual. Saf.*, **1**: 217-221.

ELLINGER, CH. (1985) Enzyme activities after *in vitro* and *in vivo* application of dichlorvos. *Biomed. Biochim. Acta*, **44**(2): 311-316.

ELLINGER, CH., KAISER, G., & HÖRING, H. (1985) [Haematological changes to rats following exposure to dichlorvos.] *Nahrung*, **29**(4): 351-355 (in German).

ELLMAN, G.L., COURTNEY, K.D., ANDRES, V., Jr, & FEATHERSTONE, R.M. (1961) A new and rapid colorimetric determination of acetylcholinesterase activity. *Biochem. Pharmacol.*, **7**: 88-95.

ENOMOTO, M.F., NAKADATE, M., NINOMIYA, K., HAYAKAWA, Y., ITO, H., IGARASHI, S., UWANUMA, Y., NAKASATO, R., & HATANAKA, J. (1981) *Studies on carcinogenicity of DDVP (2,2-dichlorovinyl dimethyl phosphate) mixed in drinking-water in rats*, Tokyo, Ministry of Health and Welfare (Cooperative Studies on Carcinogenicity Test on Mutagens) (unpublished).

EPSTEIN, S.S., ARNOLD, E., ANDREA, J., BASS, W., & BISHOP, Y. (1972) Detection of chemical mutagens by the dominant lethal assay in the mouse. *Toxicol. appl. Pharmacol.*, **23**: 288-325.

ERIKSSON, H. & FAYERSSON, Y. (1980) A reliable way of estimating cholinesterases from whole blood in the presence of anticholinesterases. *Clin. Chim. Acta*, **100**: 165-171.

ESCUDIE, E. & SALES, P. (1963) Premières expériences en Haute Volta sur le dichlorvos résiduel. *Bull. World Health Organ.*, **29**: 247-249.

FAHRIG, R. (1973) [Genetic effects of organophosphorus insecticides.] *Naturwissenschaften*, **60**(1): 50-51 (in German).

FAHRIG, R. (1974) Comparative mutagenicity studies with pesticides. In: Montesano, R. & Tomotis, L., ed. *Chemical carcinogenesis essays*, Lyons, International Agency for Research on Cancer, pp. 161-181 (IARC Scientific Publication No. 10).

FAO (1977) *FAO Specifications for plant protection products, dichlorvos and fenthion*, Rome, Food and Agriculture Organization of the United Nations.

FAO (1982) *Report of the Second Government Consultation on International Harmonization of Pesticide Registration Requirements, Rome, 11-15 October*, Rome, Food and Agriculture Organization of the United Nations.

FAO/WHO (1965a) *Evaluation of the toxicity of pesticide residues in food*, Geneva, World Health Organization (FAO PL/1965/10; WHO Food Add./26.65).

FAO/WHO (1965b) *Evaluation of the toxicity of pesticide residues in food*, Geneva, World Health Organization (FAO PL/1965/10/1; WHO Food Add./27.65).

FAO/WHO (1967a) *Pesticide residues in food. Report of the Joint Meeting on Pesticide Residues*, Geneva, World Health Organization (FAO Agricultural Studies No. 73; WHO Technical Report Series No. 370).

FAO/WHO (1967b) *Evaluation of some pesticide residues in food*, Geneva, World Health Organization (FAO PL/CP/15; WHO Food Add./67. 32).

FAO/WHO (1968a) *Pesticide residues in food. Report of the 1967 Joint Meeting on Pesticide Residues*, Geneva, World Health Organization (FAO Meeting Report No. PL/1962/M/11; WHO Technical Report Series No. 391).

FAO/WHO (1968b) *1967 Evaluation of some pesticide residues in food*, Geneva, World Health Organization (FAO PL/1967/M11/1; WHO Food Add./68.30).

FAO/WHO (1970a) *Pesticide residues in food. Report of the 1969 Joint Meeting on Pesticide Residues*, Geneva, World Health Organization (FAO Agricultural Studies No. 84; WHO Technical Report Series No. 458).

FAO/WHO (1970b) *1969 Evaluation of some pesticide residues in food*, Geneva, World Health Organization (FAO PL/1969/M/17/1; WHO Food Add./70.38).

FAO/WHO (1971a) *Pesticide residues in food. Report of the 1970 Joint Meeting on Pesticide Residues*, Geneva, World Health Organization (FAO Agricultural Studies No. 87; WHO Technical Report Series No. 474).

FAO/WHO (1971b) *1970 Evaluation of some pesticide residues in food*, Geneva, World Health Organization (AGP 1979/M/12/1; WHO Food Add./71.42).

FAO/WHO (1975a) *Pesticide residues in food. Report of the 1974 Joint Meeting on Pesticide Residues*, Geneva, World Health Organization (FAO Agricultural Studies No. 97; WHO Technical Report Series No. 574).

FAO/WHO (1975b) *1974 Evaluation of some pesticide residues in food, Geneva*, World Health Organization (AGP 1974/M/11; WHO Pesticide Residue Series No. 4).

FAO/WHO (1977a) *Pesticide residues in food. Report of the 1976 Joint Meeting of the FAO Panel of Experts on Pesticide Residues and the Environment and the WHO Expert Group on Pesticide Residues,* Geneva, World Health Organization (FAO Food and Nutrition Series No. 9; FAO Plant Production and Protection Series No. 8; WHO Technical Report Series No. 612).

FAO/WHO (1977b) *1976 Evaluations of some pesticide residues in food,* Rome, Food and Agriculture Organization of the United Nations (ADP 1977/M/14).

FAO/WHO (1978a) *Pesticide residues in food. Report of the 1977 Joint Meeting on Pesticide Residues,* Rome, Food and Agriculture Organization of the United Nations (FAO Plant Production and Protection Paper 10 Rev.).

FAO/WHO (1978b) *1977 Evaluation of some pesticide residues in food,* Rome, Food and Agriculture Organization of the United Nations (FAO Plant Production and Protection Paper 10 Suppl.).

FAO/WHO (1986) *Guide to Codex recommendations concerning pesticide residues. Part 8. Recommendations for methods of analysis of pesticide residues,* 3rd ed., Rome, Codex Committee on Pesticide Residues.

FISHBEIN, L. (1976) Potential hazards of fumigant residues. *Environ. Health Perspect.,* **14**: 39-45.

FISHBEIN, L.. (1981) Environmental sources of chemical mutagens. II. Synthetic mutagens. In: Flamm, W.G. & Mehlman, M.A., ed. *Mutagenesis: advances in modern toxicology,* Tokyo, Mishima and Kyoto, **Vol. 5**, pp. 257-348.

FISHBEIN, L. (1982) An overview of the structural features of mutagenic *S*-chlorallylthio and dithiocarbamate pesticides and trichlorfon, dichlorvos, and their metabolites. In: *Proceedings of the 3rd International Conference on Environmental Mutagens and Carcinogens, 21-27 September 1981,* Tokyo, Mishima and Kyoto, pp. 371-378.

FISCHER, G.W., SCHNEIDER, P., & SCHEUFLER, H. (1977) [Mutagenicity of dichloroacetaldehyde and 2,2-dichloro-1,1-dihydroxyethane phosphoric acid methyl ester: possible metabolites of the organophosphorus pesticide trichlorphon.] *Chem.-biol. Interact.,* **19**: 205-213 (in German).

FOLL, C.V., PANT, C.P., & LIETAERT, P.E. (1965) A large-scale field trial with dichlorvos as a residual fumigant insecticide in northern Nigeria. *Bull. World Health Organ.,* **32**: 531-550.

FOURNIER, E., DALLY, S., & CAMBIER, J. (1976) Neuropathie périphérique probablement due aux insecticides anticholinestérasiques. *Nouv. Presse méd.*, **5**(11): 718.

FRANCIS, B.M., METCALF, R.L., & HANSEN, L.G. (1985) Toxicity of organophosphorus esters to laying hens after oral and dermal administration. *J. environ. Sci. Health*, **B20**(1): 73-95.

FRANK, R., BRAUN, H.E., & FLEMING, G. (1983) Organochlorine and organophosphorus residues in fat of bovine and porcine carcasses marketed in Ontario, Canada from 1969-81. *J. food Prot.*, **46**: 893-900.

FUJITA, K., MATSUSHIMA, S., ABE, E., SASAKI, K., & KUROSAWA, K. (1977) [Examination of the effects of dichlorvos on the testis.] *Nippon Noson Igakkai Zasshi*, **26**(3): 328-329 (in Japanese).

FUJITA, Y. (1985) Studies on contact dermatitis from pesticides in tea growers. *Acta Med. Univ. Kagoshima*, **27**(1): 17-37.

FUNCKES, A.J., MILLER, S., & HAYES, W.J., Jr (1963) Initial field studies in Upper Volta with dichlorvos residual fumigant as a malaria eradication technique. *Bull. World Health Organ.*, **29**: 243-246.

GAINES, TH.B. (1969) Acute toxicity of pesticides. *Toxicol. appl. Pharmacol.*, **14**(3): 515-534.

GAINES, TH.B., HAYES, W.J., Jr, & LINDER, R.E. (1966) Liver metabolism of anticholinesterase compounds in live rats: relation to toxicity. *Nature (Lond.)*, **209**: 88-89.

GIFAP (1982) *Guidelines on pesticide residues to provide data for the registration of pesticides and the establishment of maximum residue limits elaborated by Codex Committee on Pesticide Residues*, Brussels, International Group of National Associations of Manufacturers of Agrochemical Products (Technical Monograph No. 4).

GILLENWATER, H.B., HAREIN, P.K., LOY, E.W., Jr, THOMPSON, J.F., LAUDANI, H., & EASON, G. (1971) Dichlorvos applied as a vapour in a warehouse containing packaged foods. *J. stored Prod. Res.*, **7**: 45-56.

GILLETT, J.W., HARR, J.R., LINDSTROM, F.T., MOUNT, D.A., ST. CLAIR, A.D., & WEBER, L.J. (1972) Evaluation of human health hazards on use of dichlorvos (DDVP), especially in resin strips. *Residue Rev.*, **44**: 115-159.

GILOT-DELHALLE, J., COLIZZI, A., MOUTSCHEN, J., & MOUTSCHEN-DAHMEN, M. (1983) Mutagenicity of some organophosphorus compounds at the ade6 locus of *Schizosaccharomyces pombe*. *Mutat. Res.*, **117**: 139-148.

GOH, K.S., EDMISTON, S., MADDY, K.T., & MARGETICH, S. (1986a) Dissipation of dislodgeable foliar residue for chlorpyrifos and dichlorvos treated lawn: implication for safe reentry. *Bull. environ. Contam. Toxicol.*, **37**: 33-40

GOH, K.S., EDMISTON, S., MADDY, K.T., MEINDERS, D.D., & MARGETICH, S. (1986b) Dissipation of dislodgeable foliar residue of chlorpyrifos and dichlorvos on turf. *Bull. environ. Contam. Toxicol.*, **37**: 27-32.

GOLD, R.E., HOLCSLAW, T., TUPY, D., & BALLARD, J.B. (1984) Dermal and respiratory exposure to applicators and occupants of residences treated with dichlorvos (DDVP). *J. econ. Entomol.*, **77**: 430-436.

GOTO, S. (1977) [Variation of concentrations of pesticide residues in field soil.] *J. Pestic. Sci.*, **2**: 319-321. (in Japanese, with English summary).

GOUGH, B.J. & SHELLENBERGER, T.E. (1970) *In vivo* rabbit blood cholinesterase inhibition and reactivation following organophosphate infusion. *Toxicol. appl. Pharmacol.*, **17**(1): 302.

GOUGH, B.J. & SHELLENBERGER, T.E. (1977-78) *In vivo* inhibition of rabbit whole blood cholinesterase with organophosphate inhibitors and reactivation with oximes. *Drug Chem. Toxicol.*, **1**(1): 25-43.

GRAHL, K. (1979) [The persistence of trichlorfon and dichlorvos in ponds.] *Z. Binnenfisch. DDR*, **25**(10): 312-316 (in German).

GRAHL, K., STELZER, W., & STOTTMEISTER, S. (1980) [Toxicity of butonate, trichlorfon, and dichlorvos to *Escherichia coli* and *Enterobacter aerogenes*.] *Acta hydrochim. hydrobiol.*, **8**: 19-28 (in German).

GRAHL, K., HORN, H., & HALLEBACH, R. (1981) [Effect of butonate, trichlorfon, and dichlorvos on plankton populations.] *Acta hydrochim. hydrobiol.*, **9**(2): 147-161 (in German).

GRATZ, N.G., BRACHA, P., & CARMICHAEL, A. (1963) A village- scale trial with dichlorvos as a residual fumigant insecticide in southern Nigeria. *Bull. World Health Organ.*, **29**: 251-270.

GREEN, M.H.L., BRIDGES, B.A., GRAY, W.J.H., & MOTTERSHEAD, R.P. (1973) Comparison of DNA damage caused by dichlorvos and methyl methanesulfonate in pol A and pol A^+ strains of *Escherichia coli*. *Genetics*, **74**: s100.

GREEN, M.H.L., MEDCALF, A.S.C., ARLETT, C.R., HARCOURT, S.A., & LEHMANN, A.R. (1974a) DNA strand breakage caused by dichlorvos, methyl methane-sulfonate and iodoacetamide in *Escherichia coli* and cultured Chinese hamster cells. *Mutat. Res.*, **24**(3): 365-378.

GREEN, M.H.L., MEDCALF, A.S.C., & STEVENS, S.W. (1974b) Apparent indirect DNA damage by dichlorvos and iodoacetamide in *Escherichia coli. Heredity*, **33**: 446.

GREEN, M.H.L., MURIEL, W.J., & BRIDGES, B.A. (1976) Use of a simplified fluctuation test to detect low levels of mutagens. *Mutat. Res.*, **38**(1): 33-42.

GRIFFIN, D.E., III & HILL, W.E. (1978) *In vitro* breakage of plasmid DNA by mutagens and pesticides. *Mutat. Res.*, **52**: 161-169.

GRUBNER, P. (1972) [Residue problems in the use of phosphoric acid ester insecticides in mushroom cultures.] *Nachrichtenbl. Pflanzenschutzdienst (DDR)*, **26**: 245-247 (in German).

GUNDERSON, E.C. (1981) *Sampling methods for airborne pesticides*, Washington, DC, American Chemical Society, pp. 301-315 (ACS Symposium Series No. 149).

GUPTA, A.K. & SINGH, J. (1974) Dichlorvos (DDVP) induced breaks in the salivary gland chromosomes of *Drosophila melanogaster*. *Curr. Sci.*, **43**(20): 661-662.

GUPTA, R.C., DAVE, S.K., SHAH, M.P., & KASHYAP, S.K. (1979) A monitoring study of workers handling pesticides in warehouses and godowns. *J. environ. Sci. Health*, **B14**(4): 405-416.

HALEY, T.J., FARMER, J.H., HARMON, J.R., & DOOLEY, K.L. (1975) Estimation of the LD_1 and extrapolation of the $LD_{0.1}$ for five organophosphate pesticides. *Arch. Toxicol.*, **34**: 103-109.

HANNA, P.J. & DYER, K.F. (1975) Mutagenicity of organophosphorus compounds in bacteria and *Drosophila*. *Mutat. Res.*, **28**: 405-420.

HASAN, M. & ALI, S.F. (1980) Organophosphate pesticide dichlorvos-induced increase in the rate of lipid peroxidation in the different regions of the rat brain: supporting ultra-structural findings. *Neurotoxicology*, **2**: 43-52.

HASAN, M., MAITRA, S.C., & ALI, S.F. (1979) Organophosphate pesticide DDVP-induced alterations in the rat cerebellum and spinal cord: an electron microscopic study. *Exp. Pathol.*, **17**(2): 88-94.

HASS, D.K., COLLINS, J.A., & KODAMA, J.K. (1972) Effects of orally administered dichlorvos in rhesus monkeys. *J. Am. Vet. Med. Assoc.*, **161**(6): 714-719.

HATCH, G.G., ANDERSON, T.M., HUBERT, R.A., KOURI, R.E., PUTMAN, D.L., CAMERON, J.W., NIMS, R.W., MOST, B., SPALDING, J.W., TENNANT, R.W., & SCHECHTMAN, L.M. (1986) Chemical enhancement of sa_7 virus transformation of hamster embryo cells: evaluation by interlaboratory testing of diverse chemicals. *Environ. Mutagenesis.*, **8**: 515-531.

HATTORI, K., SATO, H., TSUCHIYA, K., YAMAMOTO, N., & OGAWA, E. (1974) [Toxicological studies on the influences of chemicals to the birds. I. Oral acute toxicity and cholinesterase inhibition of three organophosphate insecticides in Japanese quail.] *Hokkaidoritsu Eisei Kenkyusho Ho*, **24**: 35-38 (in Japanese, with English summary).

HAYES, A.L., WISE, R.A., & WEIR, F.W. (1980) Assessment of occupational exposure to organophosphates in pest control operators. *Am. Ind. Hyg. Assoc. J.*, **41**(8): 568-575.

HAYES, W.J., Jr (1961) Safety of DDVP for the disinsection of aircraft. *Bull. World Health Organ.*, **24**: 629-633.

HAYES, W.J., Jr (1963) *Clinical handbook on economic poisons: emergency information for treating poisoning*, Atlanta, Georgia, US Department of Health, Education and Welfare, Public Health Service, Communicable Diseases Center (Public Health Service Publication No. 476).

HAYES, W.J., Jr (1982) Organic phosphorus pesticides. In: *Pesticides studied in man*, Baltimore, Maryland, Williams and Wilkins, pp. 343-351.

HAZELWOOD, J.C., STEFAN, G.E., & BOWEN, J.M. (1979) Motor unit irritability in beagles before and after exposure to cholinesterase inhibitors. *Am. J. vet. Res.*, **40**(6): 852-856.

HEMMINKI, K. (1983) Nucleic acid adducts of chemical carcinogens and mutagens. *Arch. Toxicol.*, **52**: 249-285.

HENRIKSSON, K., KALLELA, K., VIRTAMO, M., & PFAFFLI, P. (1971) [The toxicity of DDVP (dichlorvos) evaporated from Vapona strip.] *J. Sci. Agric. Soc. Finl.*, **43**: 187-200 (in Finnish).

HEUSER, S.G. & SCUDAMORE, K.A. (1966) A rapid method for sampling dichlorvos vapour in air. *Chem. Ind.*, **50**: 2093-2094.

HEUSER, S.G. & SCUDAMORE, K.A. (1975) A method for the assessment under standard conditions of the output of dichlorvos slow-release units used for insect control. *Analyst*, **100**: 129-135.

HILL, E.F., HEATH, R.G., SPANN, J.W., & WILLIAMS, J.D. (1975) *Lethal dietary toxicities of environmental pollutants to birds*, Washington DC, US Department of the Interior, Fish and Wildlife Service, pp. 1-51 (Special Scientific Report: Wildlife No. 191).

HINE, C.H. (1962) *90-day chronic toxicity studies of Vapona*^{R} *insecticide for dogs*, San Francisco, California, The Hine Laboratories (Unpublished Report No. 1, 1 September).

HINE, C.H. & SLOMKA, M.B. (1968) Human tolerance of the acute and subacute oral administration of a polyvinylchloride formulation of dichlorvos (V-3 and V-12). *Pharmacologist*, **10**: 222.

HINE, C.H. & SLOMKA, M.B. (1970) Human toxicity studies on polyvinyl chloride formulation of dichlorvos. *Toxicol. appl. Pharmacol.*, **17**(1): 304-305.

HODGSON, E. & CASIDA, J.E. (1962) Mammalian enzymes involved in the degradation of 2,2-dichlorovinyl dimethylphosphate. *J. agric. food Chem.*, **10**(3): 208-214.

HOLMSTEDT, B., NORDGREN, I., SANDOZ, M., & SUNDWALL, A. (1978) Metrifonate. Summary of toxicological and pharmacological information available. *Arch. Toxicol.*, **41**: 3-29.

HORIUCHI, N. & ANDO, Y. (1978) *[Photosensitivity caused by pesticides.]* (original unpublished information used as a basis for article by Horiuchi et al., 1978) (in Japanese).

HORIUCHI, N., ANDO, S., & SUZUKI, A. (1978) [Photosensitization due to pesticides.] *Nippon Noson Igakkai Zashi*, **27**(3): 450-451 (in Japanese).

HORVATH, J., HEGATH, V., & PUCHA, K. (1968) A study of the influence of cholinesterase with cattle housed in byres provided with DDVP strips. *Agrochemia*, **8**(9): 267-268.

HUNTER, C.G. (1969) *Report on initial studies of deliberate exposures to high concentrations of dichlorvos by human subjects*, Sittingbourne, Tunstall Laboratory Shell (Unpublished Report, July).

HUNTER, C.G. (1970a) *Dichlorvos: inhalational exposures with human subjects. Part 1*, Sittingbourne, Shell Research Ltd (Unpublished Report No. TLGR.0061.70).

HUNTER, C.G. (1970b) *Dichlorvos: inhalational exposures with human subjects. Part 2,* Sittingbourne, Shell Research Ltd (Unpublished Report No. TLGR.0067.70).

HUSSEY, N.W. & HUGHES, J.T. (1964) Investigations on the use of dichlorvos in the control of the mushroom phorid *Megaselia halterata* (Wood). *Ann. appl. Biol.,* **54**: 129-139.

HUTSON, D.H. & HOADLEY, E.C. (1972a) The comparative metabolism of ^{14}C-vinyl-dichlorvos in animals and man. *Arch. Toxikol.,* **30**: 9-18.

HUTSON, D.H. & HOADLEY, E.C. (1972b) The metabolism of ^{14} C-methyl-dichlorvos in the rat and mouse. *Xenobiotica,* **2**(2): 107-116.

HUTSON, D.H., BLAIR, D., HOADLEY, E.C., & PICKERING, B.A. (1971a) The metabolism of ^{14}C-Vapona^{R} in rats after administration by oral and inhalation routes. *Toxicol. appl. Pharmacol.,* **19**: 378-379.

HUTSON, D.H., HOADLEY, E.C., & PICKERING, B.A. (1971b) The metabolic fate of vinyl-1-^{14}C-dichlorvos in the rat after oral and inhalation exposure. *Xenobiotica,* **1**(6): 593-611.

HYDE, K.M., CRANDALL, J.C., KORTMAN, K.E., & MCCOY, W.K. (1978) EEG, ECG, and respiratory response to acute insecticide exposure. *Bull. environ. Contam. Toxicol.,* **19**: 47-55.

IARC (1979) *Some halogenated hydrocarbons,* Lyons, International Agency for Research on Cancer, pp. 97-127 (Monographs on the Evaluation of the Carcinogenic Risk of Chemicals to Humans, **Vol. 20**).

IRPTC (1984) *DDVP,* Geneva, International Register of Potentially Toxic Chemicals, United Nations Environment Programme (Scientific Reviews of Soviet Literature on Toxicity and Hazards of Chemicals, No. 79).

ISSHIKI, K., MIYATA, K., MATSUI, S., TSUTSUMI, M., & WATANABE, T. (1983) [Effects of post-harvest fungicides and piperonyl butoxide on the acute toxicity of pesticides in mice.] *Shokuhin Eiseigaku Zasshi,* **24**(3): 268-274 (in Japanese, with English summary).

IVEY, M.C. & CLABORN, H.V. (1969) GLC determination of dichlorvos in milk, eggs and various body tissues of cattle and chickens. *J. Assoc. Off. Anal. Chem.,* **52**(6): 1248-1251.

IWATA, Y., SUGITANI, A., & YAMADA, F. (1981) [An analytical method for organophosphorus pesticides in the onion.] *Shokuhin Eiseigaku Zasshi,* **22**: 484-489 (in Japanese, with English summary).

JAKUBOWSKA, B. & NOWAK, A. (1973) [The effect of organophosphorus and carbamate insecticides on the development of soil fungi.] *Zesz. Nauk. Akad. Roln. Szczecinie*, **39**(10): 141-150 (in Polish).

JAQUES, R. (1964) The protective effect of pyridine-2-aldoxime methiodide (P2AM), bis-(4-hydroxyimino-methyl-pyridinium-1-methyl)-ether dichloride (Toxogonin[R]) and atropine in experimental DDVP poisoning. *Helv. Physiol. Pharmacol. Acta*, **22**(3): 174-183.

JAYASURIYA, V.U., DE S. & RATNAYAKE, W.E. (1973) Screening of some pesticides on *Drosophila melanogaster* for toxic and genetic effects. *Drosophila Inf. Serv.*, **50**: 184-186.

JENSEN, J.A., FLURY, V.P., & SCHOOF, H.F. (1965) Dichlorvos vapour disinsection of aircraft. *Bull. World Health Organ.*, **32**: 175-179.

JOHNSON, M.K. (1969) The delayed neurotoxic effect of some organophosphorus compounds. Identification of the phosphorylation site as an esterase. *Biochem. J.*, **114**(4): 711-717.

JOHNSON, M.K. (1975a) The delayed neuropathy caused by some organophosphorus esters: mechanisms and challenge. *CRC Crit. Rev. Toxicol.*, **3**: 289-316.

JOHNSON, M.K. (1975b) Organophosphorus esters causing delayed neurotoxic effects. Mechanism of action and structure/ activity studies. *Arch. Toxicol.*, **34**: 259-288.

JOHNSON, M.K. (1978) The anomalous behaviour of dimethyl phosphates in the biochemical test for delayed neurotoxicity. *Arch. Toxicol.*, **41**: 107-110.

JOHNSON, M.K. (1981) Delayed neurotoxicity: do trichlorphon and/or dichlorvos cause delayed neuropathy in man or in test animals? *Acta pharmacol. toxicol.*, **49**(Suppl. 5): 87-98.

JOHNSON, R.D., MANSKE, D.D., & PODREBARAC, D.S. (1981a) Pesticide metal and other chemical residues in adult total diet samples. XII. *Pestic. monit. J.*, **15**(1): 54-69.

JOHNSON, R.D., MANSKE, D.D., NEW, D.H., & PODREBARAC, D.S. (1981b) Pesticide, heavy metal, and other chemical residues in infant and toddler total diet samples. II. August 1975 - July 1976. *Pestic. monit. J.*, **15**(1): 39-50.

JOHNSON, W.W. & FINLEY, M.T. (1980) *Handbook of acute toxicity of chemicals to fish and aquatic invertebrates*, Washington DC, US Department of the Interior, Fish and Wildlife Service (Resource Publication No. 137).

JOLLEY, W.P., STEMMER, K.L., & PFITZER, E.A. (1967) *The effects exerted upon beagle dogs during a period of two years by the introduction of Vapona*[R] insecticide into their daily diet, Cincinnati, Ohio, The Kettering Laboratory (Unpublished Report, 19 January).

KAWACHI, T., KOMATSU, T., KADA, T., ISHIDATE, M., SASAKI, M., SUGIYAMA, T., & TAZIMA, Y. (1980) Results of recent studies on the relevance of various short-term screening tests in Japan. In: G.M. Williams et al., ed. *The predictive value of short-term screening tests in carcinogenicity evaluation*, Amsterdam, Oxford, New York, Elsevier/North Holland Biomedical Press, pp. 253-267.

KENAGA, E.E. (1979) Acute and chronic toxicity of 75 pesticide to various animal species. *Down Earth*, **35**(2): 25-31

KIMBROUGH, R.D. & GAINES, T.B. (1968) Effect of organic phosphorus compounds and alkylating agents on the rat fetus. *Arch. environ. Health*, **16**: 805-808.

KIMMERLE, G. & LORKE, D. (1968) [Toxicity of insecticidal phosphoric acid esters.] *Pflanzenschutz Nachr. Bayer*, **21**(1): 111-142 (in German).

KIRKLAND, V.L. (1971) Some aspects of acute inhalation pharmacology of dichlorvos in swine. Paper presented at: *American Chemical Society for Pharmacology and Experimental Therapeutics and the Division of Medical Chemistry, Burlington, Vermont, 25 August, 1971.*

KLIGERMAN, A.D., EREXSON, G.L., & WILMER, J.L. (1985) Induction of sister-chromatid exchange (SCE) and cell-cycle inhibition in mouse peripheral blood B lymphocytes exposed to mutagenic carcinogens *in vivo*. *Mutat. Res.*, **157**: 181-187.

KNAPP, F.W. & GRADEN, A.P. (1964) Accidental exposure of dairy cows to excessive amount of dichlorvos. *J. econ. Entomol.*, **57**: 790-791.

KOBAYASHI, H., YUYAMA, A., IMAJO, S., & MATSUSAKA, N. (1980) Effects of acute and chronic administration of DDVP (dichlorvos) on distribution of brain acetylcholine in rats. *J. toxicol. Sci.*, **5**: 311-319.

KOBAYASHI, H., YUYAMA, A., & CHIBA, K.I. (1986) Cholinergic system of brain tissue in rats poisoned with the organophosphate *0,0*-demethyl *0*-(2,2-dichlorovinyl) phosphate. *Toxicol. appl. Pharmacol.*, **82**: 32-39.

KODAMA, J.K. (1960) *Technical DDVP. Acute oral administration: dogs*, Vienna, Virginia, Hazleton Laboratories (Unpublished Report, 20 January).

KODAMA, J.K. (1968) *Experimental evaluation in guinea-pigs of skin-sensitizing potential of components of formulated dichlorvos/polyvinylchloride products,* Modesto, California, Shell Development Company (Unpublished Technical Progress Report No. M-67-68).

KONISHI, Y., DENDA, A., & KITAOKA, R. (1981) *Studies on carcinogenicity of dichlorvos in B6C3FI mice,* Tokyo, Ministry of Health and Welfare (Cooperative Studies on Carcinogenicity Tests on Mutagens) (unpublished).

KRAMERS, P.G.N. & KNAAP, A.G.A.C. (1978) Absence of a mutagenic effect after feeding dichlorvos to larvae of *Drosophila melanogaster. Mutat. Res.,* **57**: 103-105.

KRAUSE, CHR., VON & KIRCHHOFF, J. (1970) [Gas chromatographic determination of organophosphate residues in market samples of fruits and vegetables.] *Dtsch. Lebensm. Rundschau.,* **66**(6): 194-199 (in German).

KRAUSE, W. (1977) Influence of DDT, DDVP, and malathion on FSH, LH, and testosterone serum levels and testosterone concentrations in testis. *Bull. environ. Contam. Toxicol.,* **18**(2): 231-242.

KRAUSE, W. & HOMOLA, S. (1972) [Influence on spermatogenesis by DDVP (dichlorvos).] *Arch. Dermatol. Forsch.,* **244**: 439-441 (in German).

KRAUSE, W. & HOMOLA, S. (1974) Alterations of the seminiferous epithelium and the Leydig cells of the rat* testis after the application of dichlorvos (DDVP). *Bull. environ. Contam. Toxicol.,* **11**(5): 429-433 (*study was performed on mice).

KRAUSE, W., HAMM, K., & WEISSMULLER, J. (1976) Damage to spermatogenesis in juvenile rat treated with DDVP and malathion. *Bull. environ. Contam. Toxicol.,* **15**(4): 458-462.

KUWABARA, K., NAKAMURA, A., & KASHIMOTO, T. (1980) Effect of petroleum oil, pesticides, PCBs, and other environmental contaminants on the hatchability of *Artemia salina* dry eggs. *Bull. environ. Contam. Toxicol.,* **25**: 69-74.

LAFONTAINE, A., AERTS, J., & JACQUES, P. (1981) [Toxicity, carcinogenic, mutagenic, and teratogenic action of dichlorvos.] *Arch. belg. Méd. soc. Hyg. Méd. Trav. Méd. lég.,* **39**(3): 159-174 (in Dutch).

LAL, R. (1982) Accumulation, metabolism, and effects of organophosphorus insecticides on microorganisms. *Adv. appl. Microbiol.,* **28**: 149-200.

LAMOREAUX, R.J. & NEWLAND, L.W. (1978) The fate of dichlorvos in soil. *Chemosphere,* **7**(10): 807-814.

LAWLEY, P.D., SHAH, S.A., & ORR, D.J. (1974) Methylation of nucleic acids by 2,2-dichlorovinyl dimethyl phosphate (dichlorvos, DDVP). *Chem.-biol. Interact.*, **8**: 171-182.

LAWS, E.R., Jr (1966) Route of absorption of DDVP after oral administration to rats. *Toxicol. appl. Pharmacol.*, **8**: 193-196.

LEARY, J.S., HIRSCH, L., LAVOR, E.M., FEICHTMEIR, E., SCHULTZ, D., KOOS, B., ROAN, C.R., FONTENOT, C., & HINE, C.H. (1971) An evaluation of the safety of No-Pest[R] strip insecticide with special reference to respiratory and dietary exposure of occupants of homes in Arizona. *Toxicol. appl. Pharmacol.*, **19**: 379.

LEARY, J.S., KEANE, W.T., FONTENOT, C., FEICHTMEIR, E.F., SCHULTZ, D., KOOS, B.A., HIRSCH, L., LAVOR, E.M., ROAN, C.C., & HINE, C.H. (1974) Safety evaluation in the home of polyvinyl chloride resin strips containing dichlorvos (DDVP). *Arch. environ. Health,* **29**: 308-314.

LEONARD, A. (1976) Heritable chromosome aberrations in mammals after exposure to chemicals. *Radiat. environ. Biophys.*, **13**: 1-8.

LEWIS, R.G. (1976) Sampling and analysis of airborne pesticides. In: Lee, R.L., ed. *Air pollution from pesticides and agricultural processes,* Cleveland, Ohio, CRC Press, pp. 51-95.

LIEBERMAN, M.T. & ALEXANDER, M. (1981) Effects of pesticides on decomposition of organic matter nitrification in sewage. *Bull. environ. Contam. Toxicol.*, **26**: 554-560.

LIEBERMAN, M.T. & ALEXANDER, M. (1983) Microbial and non-enzymatic steps in the decomposition of dichlorvos (2,2-dichlorovinyl *O,O*-dimethylphosphate). *J. agric. food Chem.*, **31**: 265-267.

LIVINGSTON, R.J. (1977) Review of current literature concerning the acute and chronic effects of pesticides on aquatic organisms. *CRC crit. Rev. environ. Control,* **7**: 325-351.

LLOYD, T.S. (1973) Accidental poisoning in birds. *Vet. Rec.*, **5 May**: 489.

LOEFFLER, J.E., DE VRIES, D.M., YOUNG, R., & PAGE, A.C. (1971) Metabolic fate of inhaled dichlorvos in pigs. *Toxicol. appl. Pharmacol.*, **19**: 378.

LOEFFLER, J.E., POTTER, J.C., SCORDELIS, S.L., HENDRICKSON, H.R., HUSTON, C.K., & PAGE, A.C. (1976) Long-term exposure of swine to a ^{14}C-dichlorvos atmosphere. *J. agric. food Chem.*, **24**(2): 367-371.

LÖFROTH, G. (1970) Alkylation of DNA by dichlorvos. *Naturwissenschaften*, **57**(8): 393-394.

LÖFROTH, G. (1978) The mutagenicity of dichloroacetaldehyde. *Z. Naturforsch.*, **33**: 783-785.

LÖFROTH, G. & WENNERBERG, R. (1974) Methylation of purines and nicotinamide in the rat by dichlorvos. *Z. Naturforsch.*, **29**: 651.

LÖFROTH, G., KIM, C.H., & HUSSAIN, S. (1969) Alkylating properties of 2,2-dichlorovinyl dimethyl phosphate: a disregarded hazard. *Environ. Mutat. Soc. Newslett.*, **2**: 21-27.

LOHS, K., FISCHER, G.W., & DEDEK, W. (1976) [Chemical-toxicological aspects of the alkylating properties of organophosphate pesticides.] *Sitzungsber. Akad. Wiss. (DDR)*, **11N**: 1-58 (in German).

LOTTI, M. & JOHNSON, M.K. (1978) Neurotoxicity of organophosphorus pesticides: predictions can be based on *in vitro* studies with hen and human enzymes. *Arch. Toxicol.*, **41**: 215-221.

LUDKE, J.L. & LOCKE, L.N. (1976) Duck deaths from accidental ingestion of anthelmintic. *Avian Dis.*, **20**(3): 607-608.

LUKE, M.A., FROBERG, J.E., DOOSE, G.M., & MASUMOTO, H.T. (1981) Improved multiresidue gas chromatographic determination of organophosphorus organonitrogen, and organohalogen pesticides in produce, using flame photometric and electrolytic conductivity detectors. *J. Assoc. Off. Anal. Chem.*, **64**(5): 1187-1195.

MACDONALD, R. (1982) *Toxicology of consumer products: the acute (4-h) inhalation toxicity of dichlorvos vapour in rats and mice*, Sittingbourne, Shell Research Ltd (Unpublished Report SBGR.82.145).

MACKLIN, A.W. & RIBELIN, W.E. (1971) The relation of pesticides to abortion in dairy cattle. *J. Am. Vet. Med. Assoc.*, **159**(12): 1743-1748.

MADDY, K.T., EDMISTON, S., & FREDRICKSON, A.S. (1981a) *Monitoring residue of DDVP in room air and on horizontal surfaces following use of a room fogger*, Sacramento, California, California Department of Food and Agriculture (Unpublished Report No. HS-897).

MADDY, K.T., SCHNEIDER, F., LOWE, J., OCHI, E., FREDRICKSON, A.S., & MARGOTICH, S. (1981b) *Vapona (DDVP) exposure potential to in mushroom houses in Ventura County, California, in 1981*, Sacramento, California, California Department of Food and Agriculture (Unpublished Report No. HS-861).

MAJEWSKI, T., PODGORSKI, W., BIALKOWSKI, Z., & TYCZKOWSKI, J. (1978) [Effects of application of different forms of DDVP to cows.] *Rocz. Nauk. Zootech.*, **5**(2): 65-74 (in Polish).

MAJEWSKI, T., PODGORSKI, W., & MICHALOWSKA, R. (1979) Retention of dichlorvos (DDVP) in rabbits. *Pol. Arch. Weter.*, **21**(2): 249-255.

MASLINSKA, D. & ZALEWSKA, Z. (1978) Effect of dichlorvos administered to the pregnant rabbits on the cholinesterase activity in the progeny. *Folia histochem. cytochem.*, **16**(4): 335-341.

MASLINSKA, D., STROSZNAJDER, J., ZALEWSKA, T., & ORLEWSKI, P. (1984) Phospholipid-protein ratio in brain of suckling rabbits treated with an organophosphorus compound. *Int. J. tissue React.*, **6**(4): 317-322.

MATHIAS, C.G.T. (1983) Persistent contact dermatitis from the insecticide dichlorvos. *Contact Dermatit.*, **9**: 217-218.

MATSUMURA, F. & BOUSH, G.M. (1968) Degradation of insecticides by a soil fungus *Trichoderm viride*. *J. econ. Entomol.*, **61**(3): 610-612.

MELNIKOV, N.N. (1971) Chemistry of pesticides. *Residue Rev.*, **36**: 310-311.

MENDOZA, C.E. (1974) Analysis of pesticides by the thin-layer chromatographic enzyme inhibition technique. Part II. *Residue Rev.*, **50**: 43-72.

MENDOZA, C.E. & SHIELDS, J.B. (1971) Esterase specificity and sensitivity to organophosphorus and carbamate pesticides: factors affecting determination by thin-layer chromatography. *J. Assoc. Off. Anal. Chem.*, **54**: 507-512.

MENZ, M., LUETKEMEIER, H., & SACHSSE, K. (1974) Long-term exposure of factory workers to dichlorvos (DDVP) insecticide. *Arch. environ. Health*, **28**: 72-76.

MESTRES, R., CHEVALLIER, CH., ESPINOZA, CL., & CORNET, R. (1977) Application du couplage chromatographie gazeuse spectrométrie de masse aux méthodes de recherche et de dosage des résidus de pesticides et de micropolluants organiques dans les matériaux de l'environnement et les matières alimentaires. *Ann. Fac. exp. Chim.*, **70**(751): 177-188.

MESTRES, R., ILLES, S., CAMPO, M., & TOURTE, J. (1979a) Développement de la méthode polyvalente d'analyse des résidus des pesticides dans les plantes et les matières alimentaires d'origine végétale. *Trav. Soc. Pharm. Montpellier*, **39**: 323-328.

MESTRES, R., ATMAWIJAYA, S., & CHEVALLIER, CH. (1979b) Méthode de recherche et de dosage des résidus de pesticides dans les produits céréaliers. I. Organochlorés, organophosphorés, pyréthrines, et pyréthrinoïdes. *Ann. Fac. exp. Chim.*, **72**: 577-589.

MICHALEK, S.M. & BROCKMAN, H.E. (1969) A test for mutagenicity of Shell "No-Pest Strip Insecticide" in *Neurospora crassa. Neurospora Newslett.*, **16**: 8.

MICHEL, H.O. (1949) An electrometric method for the determination of red blood cell and plasma cholinesterase activity. *J. lab. clin. Med.*, **34**: 1564-1568.

MILES, J.W., FETZER, L.E., & PEARCE, G.W. (1970) Collection and determination of trace quantities of pesticides in air. *Environ. Sci. Technol.*, **4**: 420-425.

MITSUI, T., OZAKI, H., KUMANO, H., & SANO, H. (1963) Insecticide determination. I. Colormetric determination of dimethyl 2,2-dichlorovinyl phosphate (DDVP). *Chem. pharm. Bull.*, **11**(5): 619-623.

MIYAMOTO, J. (1959) Non-enzymatic conversion of Dipterex into DDVP and their inhibitory action on enzymes. *Botyu-Kagaku (Sci. pestic. Control)*, **24**: 130-137.

MODAK, A.T., STAVINOHA, W.B., & WEINTRAUB, S.T. (1975) Dichlorvos and the cholinergic system: effects on cholinesterase and acetylcholine and choline contents of rat tissues. *Arch. int. Pharmacodyn.*, **217**: 293-301.

MOHN, G. (1973) *S*-methyltryptophan resistance mutations in *Escherichia coli* K12. Mutagenic activity of mono-functional alkylating agents including organophosphorus insecticides. *Mutat. Res.*, **20**: 7-15.

MORIYA, M., KATO, K., & SHIRASU, Y. (1978) Effects of cysteine and a liver metabolic activation system on the activities of mutagenic pesticides. *Mutat. Res.*, **57**: 259-263.

MORIYA, M., OHTA, T., WATANABE, K., MIYAZAWA, T., KATO, K., & SHIRASU, Y. (1983) Further mutagenicity studies on pesticides in bacterial reversion assay systems. *Mutat. Res.*, **116**: 185-216.

MORPURGO, G., BELLINCAMPI, D., GUALANDI, G., BALDINELLI, L., & SERLUPI CRESCENZI, O. (1979) Analysis of mitotic non-disjunction with *Aspergillus nidulans. Environ. Health Perspect.*, **31**: 81-95.

MOUTSCHEN-DAHMEN, J., MOUTSCHEN-DAHMEN, M., & DEGRAEVE, N. (1981) Metrifonate and dichlorvos: cytogenetic investigations. *Acta pharmacol. toxicol.*, **49**(Suppl. 5): 29-39.

MULLER, G.H. (1970) Flea collar dermatitis in animals. *J. Am. Vet. Med. Assoc.*, **157**(11): 1616-1626.

NAGY, ZS., MILE, I., & ANTONI, F. (1975) The mutagenic effect of pesticides on *Escherichia coli* WP2 try$^-$. *Acta microbiol. Acad. Sci. Hung.*, **22**: 309-314.

NAIDU, N.V., REDDY, K.S., JANARDHAN, A., & MURTHY, M.K. (1978) Toxicological investigation of dichlorvos in chicks. *Indian J. Pharmacol.*, **10**(14): 323-326.

NAKAMURA, K. & SHIBA, H. (1980) [Study on pesticide residues in fruit and vegetables.] *Bull. Saitama prefect. agric. exp. Stn*, **36**: 35-56 (in Japanese).

NARCISSE, J.K. (1967) *A potentiation study in rats of Vapona*^{R} with 26 other cholinesterase-inhibiting compounds, Menlo Park, California, Stanford Research Institute (Unpublished Report, 2 June).

NCI (1977) *Bioassay of dichlorvos for possible carcinogenicity*, Bethesda, Maryland, National Cancer Institute.

NEUWIRTH, E.A. & WHITE, T.T. (1961) Safety aspects of DDVP. *Soap chem. Spec.*, **37**(3): 95-98.

NICHOLAS, A.H., VIENNE, M., & BERGHE, H., VAN DEN (1978) Sister chromatid exchange frequencies in cultured human cells exposed to an organophosphorus insecticide: dichlorvos. *Toxicol. Lett.*, **2**(5): 271-275.

NIOSH (1979) *NIOSH Manual of analytical methods. Analytical method No. P and CAM 295*, 2nd ed., Cincinnati, Ohio, National Institute for Occupational Safety and Health, **Vol. 5** (Publication No. 79-144).

NISHIO, A. & UYEKI, E.M. (1981) Induction of sister chromatid exchanges in Chinese hamster ovary cells by organophosphorus insecticides and their oxygen analogs. *J. Toxicol. environ. Health*, **8**: 939-946.

NISHIO, A. & UYEKI, E.M. (1982) Nuclease sensitivity of methylated DNA as a probe for chromatin reconstitution by genotoxicants. *Biochem. biophys. Res. Commun.*, **107**(2): 485-491.

NORDGREN, I., BERGSTROM, M., HOLMSTEDT, B., & SANDOZ, M. (1978) Transformation and action of metrifonate. *Arch. Toxicol.*, **41**: 31-41.

NOWELL, P.T., SCOTT, C.A., & WILSON, A. (1962) Hydrolysis of neostigmine by plasma-cholinesterase. *Br. J. Pharmacol.*, **19**: 498-502.

NTP (1986) *Carcinogenicity study in rats and mice with dichlorvos*, Research Triangle Park, North Carolina, US National Toxicology Program (Unpublished data).

NTP (1987) *NTP technical report on the toxicology and carcinogenesis of dichlorvos*, Research Triangle Park, North Carolina, US National Toxicology Program (NTP-TR342).

OBA, T. & KAWABATA, G. (1962) [Application of infrared absorption spectroscopy to examination of drugs and their preparations. XIV. Determination of *O,O*-dimethyl 2,2-dichlorovinyl phosphate (DDVP) and its preparation.] *Eiseishikenjo-hokoku*, **80**: 1-3 (in Japanese, with English summary).

OGATA, H., SAITO, E., MURATA, H., SHIBAZAKI, T., & INOUE, T. (1975) [A new colorimetric method of determination of *O,O*-dimethyl 2,2-dichlorovinyl phosphate in insecticidal preparations.] *Yakugaku Zasshi*, **95**(12): 1483-1491 (in Japanese, with English summary).

OLINSKI, R., WALTER, Z., WIADERKIEWICZ, R., LUKASOVA, E., & PALECEK, E. (1980) Changes in DNA properties due to treatment with the pesticides malathion and DDVP. *Radiat. environ. Biophys.*, **18**: 65-72.

OMKAR, & SHUKLA, G.S. (1984) Alteration in carbohydrate metabolism of fresh-water prawn *Macrobianchium lamarrei* after dichlorvos exposure. *Ind. Health*, **22**: 133-136.

PACHECKA, J., SULINSKI, A., & TRACZYKIEWICZ, K. (1977) The effect of acute intoxication by dichlorvos and trichlorphon on the activities of some rat brain esterases. *Neuropathol. Polska*, **15**(1): 85-92.

PAGE, A.C., DE VRIES, D.M., YOUNG, R., & LOEFFLER, J.E. (1971) Metabolic fate of ingested dichlorvos in swine. *Toxicol. appl. Pharmacol.*, **19**: 378.

PAGE, A.C., LOEFFLER, J.E., HENDRICKSON, H.R., HUSTON, C.K., & DEVRIES, D.M. (1972) Metabolic fate of dichlorvos in swine. *Arch. Toxikol.*, **30**: 19-27.

PAIK, S.G. & LEE, S.Y. (1977) Genetic effects of pesticides in the mammalian cells. I. Induction of micronucleus. *Korean J. Zool.*, **20**(1): 19-28.

PENA CHAVARRIA, A., SWARTZWELDER, J.C., VILLAREJOS, V.M., KOTCHER, E., & ARGUEDAS, J. (1969) Dichlorvos: an effective broad-spectrum anthelmintic. *Am. J. trop. Med. Hyg.*, **18**(6): 907-911.

PEROCCO, P. & FINI, A. (1980) Damage by dichlorvos of human lymphocyte DNA. *Tumori*, **66**: 425-430.

PLESTINA, R. (1984) *Prevention, diagnosis, and treatment of insecticide poisoning*, Geneva, World Health Organization (WHO Report No. VBC/84.889).

PODREBARAC, D.S. (1984) Pesticide, heavy metals, and other chemical residues in infant and toddler total diet samples. IV. October 1977 - September 1978. *J. Assoc. Off. Anal. Chem.*, **67**(1): 166-175.

POTTER, J.C., LOEFFLER, J.E., COLLINS, R.D., YOUNG, R., & PAGE, A.C. (1973a) Carbon-14 balance and residues of dichlorvos and its metabolites in pigs dosed with dichlorvos-^{14}C. *J. agric. food Chem.*, **21**(2): 163-166.

POTTER, J.C., BOYER, A.C., MARXMILLER, R.E., YOUNG, R., & LOEFFLER, J.E. (1973b). Radioisotope residues and residues of dichlorvos and its metabolites in pregnant sows and their progeny dosed with dichlorvos-^{14}C or dichlorvos-^{36}Cl formulated as PVC pellets. *J. agric. food Chem.*, **21**(4): 734-738.

PURSHOTTAM, T. & KAVEESHWAR, U. (1979) Effect of diet on dichlorovinyl dimethyl phosphate toxicity in rats. *Aviat. Space environ. Med.*, **50**(6): 581-584.

PURSHOTTAM, T. & SRIVASTAVA, R.K. (1984) Effect of high-fat and high-protein diets on toxicity of parathion and dichlorvos. *Arch. environ. Health*, **39**(6): 425-430.

PYM, R.A.E., SINGH, G., GILBERT, W.S., ARMSTRONG, J.P., & MCCLEARY, B.V. (1984) Effects of dichlorvos, maldison, and pirimiphos-methyl on food consumption, egg production, egg and tissue residues, and plasma acetylcholinesterase inhibition in layer strain hens. *Aust. J. exp. Agric. anim. Husb.*, **24**: 83-92.

QUARTERMAN, K.D., LOTTE, M., & SCHOOF, H.F. (1963) Initial field studies in Upper Volta with dichlorvos residual fumigant as a malaria eradication technique. *Bull. World Health Organ.*, **29**: 231-235.

RADELEFF, R.D. & WOODARD, G.T. (1957) The toxicity of organic phosphorus insecticides to livestock. *J. Am. Vet. Med. Assoc.*, **130**: 215-216.

RAHMATULLAH, M., JAHAN, R., CHOWDHURY, A.A., FARUK, A.B.M., & CHOWDHURY, M.S.K. (1978) Effect of organophosphorus insecticides on fermentation processes in *Aspergillus niger*. *J. ferment. Technol.*, **56**: 169-172.

RAMEL, C. (1981) Does dichlorvos constitute a genotoxic hazard? In: Kappas, A., ed. *Progress in environmental mutagenesis and carcinogenesis*, Amsterdam, Oxford, New York, Elsevier Science Publishers, pp. 69-78 (Progress in Mutation Research, **Vol.** 2.).

RAMEL, C., DRAKE, J., & SUGIMURA, T. (1980) An evaluation of the genetic toxicity of dichlorvos. *Mutat. Res.*, **76**: 297-309.

RASMUSSEN, W.A., JENSEN, J.A., STEIN, W.J., & HAYES, W.J. (1963) Toxicological studies of DDVP for disinsection of aircraft. *Aerosp. Med.*, **34**(7): 593-600.

RATH, S. & MISRA, B.N. (1979a) Relative toxicity of dichlorvos (DDVP) to *Tilapia mossambica* Peters of 3 different age groups. *Exp. Gerontol.*, **14**: 307-309.

RATH, S. & MISRA, B.N. (1979b) Sub-lethal effects of dichlorvos (DDVP) on respiratory metabolism of *Tilapia mossambica* of 3 age groups. *Exp. Gerontol.*, **14**: 37-41.

RATH, S. & MISRA, B.N. (1980) Pigment disperson in *Tilapia mossambica* Peters exposed to dichlorvos (DDVP). *Curr. Sci.*, **49**(23): 907-909.

RATH, S. & MISRA, B.N. (1981) Toxicological effects of dichlorvos (DDVP) on brain and liver acetylcholinesterase (AChE) activity of *Tilapia mossambica* Peters. *Toxicology*, **19**: 239-245.

RAUWS, A.G. & LOGTEN, M.J., VAN (1973) The influence of dichlorvos from strips or sprays on cholinesterase activity in chicken. *Toxicology*, **1**: 29-41.

REECE, R.L. (1982) Observations on the accidental poisoning of birds by organophosphate insecticides and other toxic substances. *Vet. Rec.*, **111**(20): 453-455.

REEVES, J.D., DRIGGERS, D.A., & KILEY, V.A. (1981) Household insecticide associated aplastic anaemia and acute leukaemia in children. *Lancet*, **8 August**: 300-301.

REINER, E. & PLESTINA, R. (1979) Regeneration of cholinesterase activities in humans and rats after inhibition by *O,O*-dimethyl-2,2-dichlorovinyl phosphate. *Toxicol. appl. Pharmacol.*, **49**: 451-454.

RIDER, J.A., MOELLER, H.C., & PULETTI, E.J. (1967) Continuing studies on anticholinesterase effects of methyl parathion, initial studies with Guthion, and determination of incipient toxicity level of dichlorvos in humans. *Fed. Proc.*, **26**: 427.

RIDER, J.A., MOELLER, H.C., PULETTI, E.J., & SWADER, J. (1968) Studies on the anticholinesterase effects of methyl parathion, guthion, dichlorvos, and gardona in human subjects. *Fed. Proc.*, **27**: 597.

ROSENBERG, A., LIEBERMAN, M.T., & ALEXANDER, M. (1979) *Microbial degradation of pesticides*, Springfield, Virginia, US National Technical Information Service (PB 79-123156).

ROSENKRANZ, H.S. (1973) Preferential effect of dichlorvos (Vapona[R]) on bacteria deficient in DNA polymerase. *Cancer Res.*, **33**: 458-459.

ROSENKRANZ, H.S. & LEIFER, Z. (1980) Determining the DNA-modifying activity of chemicals using DNA polymerase-deficient *Escherichia coli*. In: de Serres, F.J. & Hollander, A., ed. *Chemical mutagens: principles and methods for their detection*, New York, Plenum Press, Vol. **6**, pp. 109-147.

ROSENKRANZ, H.S. & ROSENKRANZ, S. (1972) Reaction of DNA with phosphoric acid esters: gasoline additive and insecticides. *Experientia (Basel)*, **28**(4): 386-387.

SAGNER, G. & SCHONDUBE, M. (1982) [Determination and toxicological appraisal of indoor concentrations of dichlorvos after the application of spraying products.] *Schriftenr. Ver. Wasser Boden Lufthyg.*, **53**: 359-368 (in German).

SAKAMA, K. & NISHIMURA, M. (1977) [Studies on inhalation toxicity of organic phosphorus insecticides. II. Approach to establishment of threshold limit value.] *Jpn. J. ind. Health*, **19**: 357-358 (in Japanese).

SASINOVICH, L.M. (1968) [Substantiation of the maximum permissible concentration of DDVP in the air of the working zone.] *Gig. i Sanit.*, **33**(12): 35-39 (in Russian).

SASINOVICH, L.M. (1970) [Toxicology of dimethyldichlorovinyl phosphate and hygienic characteristics of its use.] *Gig. Primen. Toksikol. Pestits. Klin. Otravl.*, **8**: 297-307 (in Russian).

SCHAFER, E.W. (1972) The acute oral toxicity of 369 pesticidal, pharmaceutical, and other chemicals to wild birds. *Toxicol. appl. Pharmacol.*, **21**: 315-330.

SCHAFER, E.W., Jr & BRUNTON, R.B. (1979) Indicator bird species for toxicity determinations: is the technique usable in test method development? In: Beck, J.R., ed. *Vertebrate pest control and management materials*, Philadelphia, Pennsylvania, American Society for Testing and Materials, pp. 157-168 (ASTM STP 680).

SCHMIDT, G., SCHMIDT, M., & NENNER, M. (1975) Inhibition of acetylcholinesterase in the bronchial system of rats caused by inhalation of dichlorvos (DDVP). *Naunyn Schmiedeberg Arch. Pharmacol.*, **287**(Suppl.): R97.

SCHMIDT, G., SCHMIDT, M., NENNER, M., & VETTERLEIN, F. (1979) Effects of dichlorvos (DDVP) inhalation on the activity of acetylcholinesterase in the bronchial tissue of rats. *Arch. Toxicol.*, **42**: 191-198.

SCHOOF, H.F., JENSEN, J.A., PORTER, J.E., & MADDOCK, D.R. (1961) Disinsection of aircraft with a mechanical dispenser of DDVP vapour. *Bull. World Health Organ.*, **24**: 623-628.

SCHULTZ, D.R., MARXMILLER, R.L., & KOOS, B.A. (1971) Residue determination of dichlorvos and related metabolites in animal tissue and fluids. *J. agric. food Chem.*, **19**(6): 1238-1243.

SCHULZE, H.D. (1979) [Current problems of pest control with dichlorvos in hospital.] *Z. gesamte Hyg.*, **25**(5): 421-425 (in German).

SCHWETZ, B.A., IOSET, H.D., LEONG, B.K.J., & STAPLES, R.E. (1979) Teratogenic potential of dichlorvos given by inhalation and gavage to mice and rabbits. *Teratology*, **20**: 383-388.

SEGERBÄCK, D. (1981) Estimation of genetic risks of alkylating agents. V. Methylation of DNA in the mouse by DDVP (2,2-dichlorovinyl dimethylphosphate). *Hereditas*, **94**: 73-76.

SEGERBÄCK, D. & EHRENBERG, L. (1981) Alkylating properties of dichlorvos (DDVP). *Acta pharmacol. toxicol.*, **49**(Suppl. 5): 56-66.

SERA, K., MATSUNAGA, A., MURAKAMI, A., SATO, I., YAMASHITA, K., & YOSHIMORI, H. (1959) Qualitative analysis of organic phosphorus color reactions and simple detection. *Kumamoto med. J.*, **12**(3): 193-213.

SHAFIK, M.T., BRADWAY, D., & ENOS, H.F. (1971) A method for confirmation of organophosphorus compounds at the residue level. *Bull. environ. Contam. Toxicol.*, **6**(1): 55-66.

SHELLENBERGER, T.E. (1980) Organophosphorus pesticide inhibition of cholinesterase in laboratory animals and man and effects of oxime reactivators. *J. environ. Sci. Health*, **B15**(6): 795-822.

SHELLENBERGER, T.E., NEWELL, G.W., OKAMOTO, S.S., & SARROS, A. (1965) Response of rabbit whole blood cholinesterase *in vivo* after continuous intravenous infusion and percutaneous application of dimethyl organophosphate inhibitors. *Biochem. Pharmacol.*, **14**: 943-952.

SHERMAN, M. & ROSS, E. (1961) Acute and subacute toxicity of insecticides to chicks. *Toxicol. appl. Pharmacol.*, **3**: 521-533.

SHINKAJI, N. & ADACHI, T. (1978) [The effect of certain pesticides on the predaceous mite *Amblyseius longispinosus* (Evans) (Acarina: Phytoseiidae).] *Akitsu*, **2**: 99-108 (in Japanese, with English tables).

SHINODA, H., ITO, K., MATSUNAGA, T., TAKADA, T., & NOMURA, T. (1972) Two suicides by acute pesticide intoxication. *J. Jpn. Assoc. Rural Med.*, **21**: 242-249 (in Japanese).

SHIRASU, Y., MORIYA, M., KATO, K., FURUHASHI, A., & KADA, T. (1976) Mutagenicity screening of pesticides in the microbial system. *Mutat. Res.*, **40**: 19-30.

SHOOTER, K.V. (1975) Assays for phosphotriester formation in the reaction of bacteriophage R_{17} with a group of alkylating agents. *Chem.-biol. Interact.*, **11**: 575-588.

SLOMKA, M.B. & HINE, C.H. (1981) Clinical pharmacology of dichlorvos. *Acta pharmacol. toxicol.*, **49**(Suppl. 5): 105-108.

SMITH, P.W., MERTENS, H., LEWIS, M.F., FUNKHOUSER, G.E., HIGGINS, E.A., CRANE, C.R., SANDERS, D.C., ENDECOTT, B.R., & FLUX, M. (1972) Toxicology of dichlorvos at operational aircraft cabin altitudes. *Aerosp. Med.*, **43**(5): 473-478.

SNOW, D.H. & WATSON, A.D.J. (1973) The acute toxicity of dichlorvos in the dog. I. Clinical observations and clinical pathology. *Aust. vet. J.*, **49**: 113-119.

SOBELS, F.H. & TODD, N.K. (1979) Absence of a mutagenic effect of dichlorvos on *Drosophila melanogaster*. *Mutat. Res.*, **67**: 89-92.

STANTON, H.C., ALBERT, J.R., & MERSMANN, H.J. (1979) Studies on the pharmacology and safety of dichlorvos in pigs and pregnant sows. *Am. J. vet. Res.*, **40**(3): 315-320.

STAVINOHA, W.B., MODAK, A.T., & WEINTRAUB, S.T. (1976) Rate of accumulation of acetylcholine in discrete regions of the rat brain after dichlorvos treatment. *J. Neurochem.*, **27**: 1375-1378.

STEIN, W.J., MILLER, S., & FETZER, L.E., Jr (1966) Studies with dichlorvos residual fumigant as a malaria eradication technique in Haiti. III. Toxicological studies. *Am. J. trop. Med. Hyg.*, **15**(5): 672-675.

STERNBERG, S.S. (1979) The carcinogenesis, mutagenesis, and teratogenesis of insecticides. Review of studies in animals and man. *Pharmacol. Ther.*, **6**: 147-166.

STEVENSON, D.E. & BLAIR, D. (1969) *A preliminary report on the inhalation toxicity of high concentrations of dichlorvos,* Sittingbourne, Shell Research Ltd (Unpublished Report TLGR.0024.69).

STEVENSON, D.E. & BLAIR, D. (1977) The uptake of dichlorvos during long-term inhalation studies. *Proc. Eur. Soc. Toxicol.*, **18**: 215-217.

STOERMER, D. (1985) [Occupational contact dermatitis from the pesticide dichlorvos.] *Dermatol. Monatsschr.*, **171**(4): 245-249 (in German).

TEICHERT, K., SZYMCZYK, T., CONSOLO, S., & LADINSKY, H. (1976) Effect of acute and chronic treatment with dichlorvos on rat brain cholinergic parameters. *Toxicol. appl. Pharmacol.*, **35**: 77-81.

TERAYAMA, K., HONMA, H., & KAWARABAYASHI, T. (1978) Toxicity of heavy metals and insecticides on slime mold *Physarum polycephalum. J. toxicol. Sci.*, **3**: 293-304.

TESSARI, J.D. & SPENCER, D.L. (1971) Air sampling for pesticides in the human environment. *J. Assoc. Off. Anal. Chem.*, **54**(6): 1376-1382.

TEZUKA, H., ANDO, N., SUZUKI, R., TERAHATA, M., MORIYA, M., & SHIRASU, Y. (1980) Sister chromatid exchanges and chromosomal aberrations in cultured Chinese hamster cells treated with pesticides positive in microbial reversion assays. *Mutat. Res.*, **78**: 177-191.

THOMAS, T.C. & NISHIOKA, Y.A. (1985) Sampling of airborn pesticides using chromosorb-102. *Bull. environ. Contam. Toxicol.*, **35**: 460-465.

THORPE, E., WILSON, A.B., DIX, K.M., & BLAIR, D. (1972) Teratological studies with dichlorvos vapour in rabbits and rats. *Arch. Toxicol.*, **30**(1): 29-38.

TIMMONS, E.M., CHAKLOS, R.J., BANNISTER, T.M., & KAPLAN, H.M. (1975) Dichlorvos effects on estrous cycle onset in the rat. *Lab. anim. Sci.*, **25**(1): 45-47.

TRACY, R.L., WOODCOCK, J.G., & CHODROFF, S. (1960) Toxicological aspects of 2,2'-dichlorovinyl dimethylphosphate (DDVP) in cows, horses, and white rats. *J. econ. Entomol.*, **53**(4): 593-601.

TUCKER, R.K. & CRABTREE, D.G. (1970) *Handbook of toxicity of pesticides to wildlife,* Washington DC, US Department of the Interior, Fish and Wildlife Service, 43 pp (Resource Publication No. 84).

UEDA, K., SHIYO, K., MORI, T., KITAHARA, E., & URAGAMI, S. (1959) [Effects of DDVP on man.] *J. Jpn. Public Hyg. Assoc.*, **6**: 315 (in Japanese).

UEDA, K., SHIYO, K., IIZUKA, Y., KITAHARA, E., & OHASHI, A. (1960) [The toxicity of organic phosphate "DDVP" for small animals and man.] *Igaku Seibutsugaku (Med. Biol.)*, **57**(3): 98-101 (in Japanese).

ULLMANN, L., PHILLIPS, J., & SACHSSE, K. (1979) Cholinesterase surveillance of aerial applicators and allied workers in the Democratic Republic of the Sudan. *Arch. environ. Contam. Toxicol.*, **8**: 703-712.

VADHVA, P. & HASAN, M. (1986) Organophosphate dichlorvos induced dose-related differential alterations in lipid levels and lipid peroxidation in various regions of the fish brain and spinal cord. *J. environ. Sci. Health*, **B21**(5): 413-424.

VAN DIJK, L.P. & VISWESWARIAH, K. (1975) Pesticides in air: sampling methods. *Residue Rev.*, **55**: 91-134.

VAN RAALTE, H.G.S. & JANSEN, J.D. (1981) Household insecticides and the blood. *Lancet*, **10 October**: 811.

VASHKOV, V.I., VOLKOVA, A.P., TSETLIN, V.M., & YANKOVSKII, E.Y. (1966) [Assessment of the use of dimethyldichlorovinyl phosphate (DDVP) in the insecticide mixture.] *Gig. i Sanit.*, **9**: 15-17 (in Russian).

VASILESCU, C. & FLORESCU, A. (1980) Clinical and electrophysiological study of neuropathy after organophosphorus compounds poisoning. *Arch. Toxicol.*, **43**: 305-315.

VERMA, S.R. & TONK, I.P. (1984) Biomonitoring of the contamination of water by a sublethal concentration of pesticides. A system analysis approach. *Acta hydrochim. hydrobiol.*, **12**(4): 399-499.

VERMA, S.R., RANI, S., BANSAL, S.K., & DALELA, R.C. (1980) Effects of the pesticides thiotox, dichlorvos, and carbofuran on the test fish *Mystus vittatus*. *Water Air Soil Pollut.*, **13**(2): 229-234.

VERMA, S.R., RANI, S., BANSAL, S.K., & DALELA, R.C. (1981a) Evaluation of the comparative toxicity of thiotox, dichlorvos, and carbofuran to two fresh water teleosts *Ophiocephalus punctatus* and *Mystus vittatus*. *Acta hydrochem. hydrobiol.*, **9**(2): 119-129.

VERMA, S.R., RANI, S., & DALELA, R.C. (1981b) Isolated and combined effects of pesticides on serum transaminases in *Mystus vittatus* (African catfish). *Toxicol. Lett.*, **8**: 67-71.

VERMA, S.R., RANI, S., & DALELA, R.C. (1981c) Pesticide-induced physiological alterations in certain tissues of a fish *Mystus vittatus*. *Toxicol. Lett.*, **9**: 327-332.

VERMA, S.R., TONK, I.P., & DALELA, R.C. (1981d) Determination of the maximum acceptable toxicant concentration (MATC) and the safe concentration for certain aquatic pollutants. *Acta hydrochim. hydrobiol.*, **9**(3): 247-254.

VERMA, S.R., BANSAL, S.K., GUPTA, A.K., PAL, N., TYAGI, A.K., BHATNAGAR, M.C., KUMAR, V., & DALELA, R.C. (1982a) Bioassay trials with twenty-three pesticides to a fresh water teleost *Saccobranchus fossilis*. *Water Res.*, **16**: 525-529.

VERMA, S.R., RANI, S., & DALELA, R.C. (1982b) Indicators of stress induced by pesticides in *Mystus vittatus:* haematological parameters. *Indian J. environ. Health*, **24**(1): 58-64.

VERMA, S.R., RANI, S., TONK, I.P., & DALELA, R.C. (1983) Pesticide-induced dysfunction in carbohydrate metabolism in three fresh water fishes. *Environ. Res.*, **32**: 127-133.

VERMA, S.R., RANI, S., & DALELA, R.C. (1984) Effects of pesticides and their combinations on three serum phosphatases of *Mystus vittatus*. *Water Air Soil Pollut.*, **21**: 9-14.

VOGIN, E.E., CARSON, S., & SLOMKA, M.B. (1971) Teratology studies with dichlorvos in rabbits. *Toxicol. appl. Pharmacol.*, **19**: 377-378.

VOOGD, C.E., JACOBS, J.J.J.A.A., & STEL, J.J., VAN DER (1972) On the mutagenic action of dichlorvos. *Mutat. Res.*, **16**: 413-416.

VOSS, G. & SACHSSE, K. (1970) Red cell and plasma cholinesterase activities in microsamples of human and animal blood determined simultaneously by a modified acetylthiocholine/DNTB procedure. *Toxicol. appl. Pharmacol.*, **16**: 764-772.

VRBOVSKY, L., SELECKY, FR.V., & ROSIVAL, L. (1959) [Toxicological and pharmacological studies with phosphorester insecticides.] *Naunyn Schmiedeberg Arch. Pharmacol.*, **236**: 202-204 (in German).

WADIA, R.S., SHINDE, S.N., & VAIDYA, (1985) Delayed neurotoxicity after an episode of poisoning with dichlorvos. *Neurology (India)*, **33**: 247-253.

WAGNER, R. & HOYER, J. (1975) [Method of determining workplace concentrations and on occupational hygiene conditions during thermal fogging atomization of pesticides in the greenhouse.] *Z. gesamte Hyg.*, **21**(1): 18-20 (in German).

WALKER, A.I.T., BLAIR, D., STEVENSON, D.E., & CHAMBERS, P.L. (1972) An inhalational toxicity study with dichlorvos. *Arch. Toxikol.*, **30**: 1-7.

WARD, F.P. & GLICKSBERG, C.L. (1971) Effects of dichlorvos on blood cholinesterase activity in dogs. *J. Am. Vet. Med. Assoc.*, **158**(4): 457-461.

WATANABE, H., SHIRAI, O., & EBATA, N. (1976) A case report of organophosphorus insecticide (DDVP) intoxication with respiratory intensive care. *Pestic. Abstr.*, **9**(2): 94-95.

WEISBURGER, E.K. (1982) Carcinogenicity tests on pesticides. In: Chambers, J.E. & Yarbrough, J.D., ed. *Effects of chronic exposures to pesticides on animal systems*, New York, Raven Press, pp. 165-176.

WENNERBERG, R. & LOFROTH, G. (1974) Formation of 7-methyl- guanine by dichlorvos in bacteria and mice. *Chem.-biol. Interact.*, **8**: 339-348.

WHITEHEAD, C.C. (1971) The effects of pesticides on production in poultry. *Vet. Rec.*, **30 January**: 114-117.

WHO (1978) *Spectrophotometric kit for measuring cholinesterase activity*, Geneva, World Health Organization (Report VBC/78.692).

WHO/FAO (1975-86) *Data sheets on pesticides*, Geneva, World Health Organization (VBC).

WHO (1985) Technical dichlorvos. In: *Specifications for pesticides used in public health*, 6th ed., Geneva, World Health Organization, pp. 163-174 (WHO/SIT/16.R2).

WHO (1986a) *The WHO recommended classification of pesticides by hazard and guidelines to classification 1986-87*, Geneva, World Health Organization, p. 11 (Report VBC/86.1 Rev.1)

WHO (1986b) *Environmental Health Criteria 63: organophosphorus insecticides: a general introduction*, Geneva, World Health Organization, 181 pp.

WILD, D. (1973) Chemical induction of streptomycin-resistant mutations in *Escherichia coli*. Dose and mutagenic effects of dichlorvos and methyl methanesulfonate. *Mutat. Res.*, **19**: 33-41.

WILD, D. (1975) Mutagenicity studies on organophosphorus insecticides. *Mutat. Res.*, **32**: 133-150.

WILDEMAUWE, C., LONTIE, J.F., SCHOOFS, L., & LAREBEKE, N., VAN (1983) The mutagenicity in procaryotes of insecticides, acaricides, and nematicides. *Residue Rev.*, **89**: 129-178.

WILLIAMS, P.P. (1977) Metabolism of synthetic organic pesticides by anaerobic microorganisms. *Residue Rev.*, **66**: 102.

WILSON, A.B. & DIX, K.M. (1973) *Toxicity studies on dichlorvos: one month inhalational exposure of rats to dichloroacetaldehyde*, Sittingbourne, Shell Research Ltd (Unpublished Report TLGR.0017.73).

WITHERUP, S., STEMMER, K.L., & CALDWELL, J.S. (1964) *The effects upon rats of being fed on diets containing Vapona*[R] insecticide, Cincinnati, Ohio, The Kettering Laboratory (Unpublished Report, 1 July).

WITHERUP, S., CALDWELL, J.S., & HULL, L. (1965) *The effects exerted upon the fertility of rats and upon the viability of their offspring by the introduction of Vapona*[R] insecticide into their diets, Cincinatti, Ohio, The Kettering Laboratory (Unpublished Report, 12 April).

WITHERUP, S., STEMMER, K.L., & PFITZER, E.A. (1967) *The effects exerted upon rats during a period of two years by the introduction of Vapona*[R] insecticide into their daily diets, Cincinnati, Ohio, The Kettering Laboratory (Unpublished Report, 14 February).

WITHERUP, S., JOLLEY, W.J., STEMMER, K., & PFITZER, E.A. (1971) Chronic toxicity studies with 2,2-dichlorovinyl dimethyl phosphate (DDVP) in dogs and rats including observations on rat reproduction. *Toxicol. appl. Pharmacol.*, **19**: 377.

WITTER, R.F. (1960) Effects of DDVP aerosols on blood cholinesterase of fogging machine operators. *Am. Med. Assoc. Arch. Ind. Health*, **21**: 7-9.

WITTER, R.F., GAINES, T.B., SHORT, J.G., SEDLAK, V.A., & MADDOCK, D.R. (1961) Studies on the safety of DDVP for the disinsection of commercial aircraft. *Bull. World Health Organ.*, **24**: 635-642.

WOOD, A.B. & KANAGASABAPATHY, L. (1983) Evaluation of inexpensive thin layer chromatographic procedures for the estimation of some organophosphorus and carbamate insecticide residues in fruit and vegetables. *Pestic. Sci.*, **14**: 108-118.

WOODER, M.F. & CREEDY, C.L. (1979) *Studies on the effects of dichlorvos on the integrity of rat liver DNA in vivo*, Sittingbourne, Shell Research Ltd (Unpublished Report TLGR.79.089).

WOODER, M.F. & WRIGHT, A.S. (1981) Alkylation of DNA by organophosphorus pesticides. *Acta pharmacol. toxicol.*, **49**(Suppl. 5): 51-55.

WOODER, M.F., WRIGHT, A.S., & KING, L.J. (1977) *In vivo* alkylation studies with dichlorvos at practical use concentrations. *Chem.-biol. Interact.*, **19**: 25-46.

WOODER, M.F., WRIGHT, A.S., & STEVENSON, D.E. (1978) Studies on the *in vivo* reactivity of methylating agents for mammalian DNA in relation to the assessment of genetic risk. *Proc. Int. Congr. Toxicol.*, **1**: 505.

WORTHING, C.R. & WALKER, S.B. (1983) *Pesticide manual*, 7th ed., Croydon, British Crop Protection Council.

WRATHALL, A.E., WELLS, D.E., & ANDERSON, P.H. (1980) Effect of feeding dichlorvos to sows in mid-pregnancy. *Zbl. Vet. Med.* **A27**: 662-668.

WRIGHT, C.G. & LEIDY, R.B. (1980) Air samples in vehicles and buildings turn up only very low levels of organic phosphate insecticides. *Pest Control*, **48**(7): 22-26, 68.

WRIGHT, A.S., HUTSON, D.H., & WOODER, M.F. (1979) The chemical and biochemical reactivity of dichlorvos. *Arch. Toxicol.*, **42**: 1-18.

XING-SHU, H. (1983) Preventing chemical damage to germ cells. *Am. Ind. Hyg. Assoc. J.*, **44**: 699-703.

YAMANE, S., KINO, A., & TESHIMA, S. (1974) Histochemical demonstration of cholinesterase activity in tissues of the carp and effect of DDVP on its activity *in situ*. *Acta histochem. cytochem.*, **7**(2): 167-174.

YAMANOI, F. (1980) [Effect of insecticides on the progeny in the silkworm *Bombyx mori*. I. Effect of organophosphorus insecticides on egg laying and their hatching.] *Nippon Sanshigaku Zasshi*, **49**(5): 434-439 (in Japanese).

YAMASHITA, K. (1960) Studies on organic phosphorus. I. Toxicity of dipterex and its vinyl derivative (DDVP). *Kumamoto med. J.*, **13**(4): 273-279.

YAMASHITA, K. (1961) Studies on organic phosphorus dipterex. III. Detection and discrimination of dipterex and its vinyl derivative (DDVP). *Kumamoto med. J.*, **14**(1): 13-25.

YAMASHITA, K. (1962) Toxicity of dipterex and its vinyl derivative (DDVP). *Ind. Med. Surg.*, **31**: 170-173.

ZALEWSKA, Z., RAKOWSKA, I., MATRASZEK, G., & SITKIEWICZ, D. (1977) Effect of dichlorvos on some enzyme activities of the rat brain during postnatal development. I. Cholinesterases. *Neuropathol. Polska,* **15**(2): 255-262.

ZAVON, M.R. & KINDEL, E.A., Jr (1966) Potential hazard in using dichlorvos insecticide resin. *Adv. Chem. Ser.,* **60**: 177-186.

ZELMAN, I.B. (1977) [Pathomorphology on the rat brain after experimental intoxication with the phosphororganic pesticide dichlorvos (DDVP).] *Neuropathol. Polska,* **15**(4): 515-522 (in Polish).

ZELMAN, I.B. & MAJDECKI, T. (1979) [Ultrastructural changes in rat brain following organophosphate insecticide dichlorvos (DDVP) intoxication.] *Neuropathol. Polska,* **17**(3): 443-453 (in Polish).

ZOTOV, V.M., SVIRIN, J.N., & PRUCAKOVA, R.M. (1977) [The development of health regulations for occupational exposure in greenhouses treated with chemical pesticides.] *Gig. Tr. prof. Zabol.,* **3**: 49-50 (in Russian).

Other titles available in the ENVIRONMENTAL HEALTH CRITERIA series (continued):

44. Mirex
45. Camphechlor
46. Guidelines for the Study of Genetic Effects in Human Populations
47. Summary Report on the Evaluation of Short-term Tests for Carcinogens (Collaborative Study on *In Vitro* Tests)
48. Dimethyl Sulfate
49. Acrylamide
50. Trichloroethylene
51. Guide to Short-term Tests for Detecting Mutagenic and Carcinogenic Chemicals
52. Toluene
53. Asbestos and Other Natural Mineral Fibres
54. Ammonia
55. Ethylene Oxide
56. Propylene Oxide
57. Principles of Toxicokinetic Studies
58. Selenium
59. Principles for Evaluating Health Risks from Chemicals During Infancy and Early Childhood: The Need for a Special Approach
60. Principles and Methods for the Assessment of Neurotoxicity Associated With Exposure to Chemicals
61. Chromium
62. 1,2-Dichloroethane
63. Organophosphorus Insecticides - A General Introduction
64. Carbamate Pesticides - A General Introduction
65. Butanols - Four Isomers
66. Kelevan
67. Tetradifon
68. Hydrazine
69. Magnetic Fields
70. Principles for the Safety Assessment of Food Additives and Contaminants in Food
71. Pentachlorophenol
72. Principles of Studies on Diseases of Suspected Chemical Etiology and Their Prevention
73. Phosphine and Selected Metal Phosphides
74. Diaminotoluenes
75. Toluene Diisocyanates
76. Thiocarbamate Pesticides - A General Introduction
77. Man-made Mineral Fibres
78. Dithiocarbamate Pesticides - A General Introduction